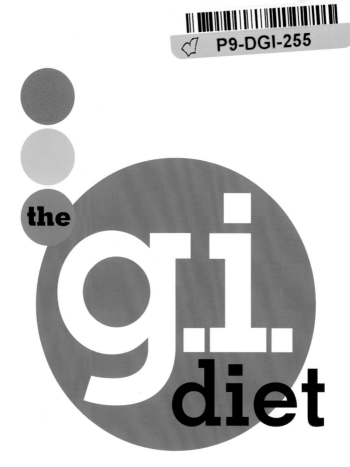

the g.i. diet

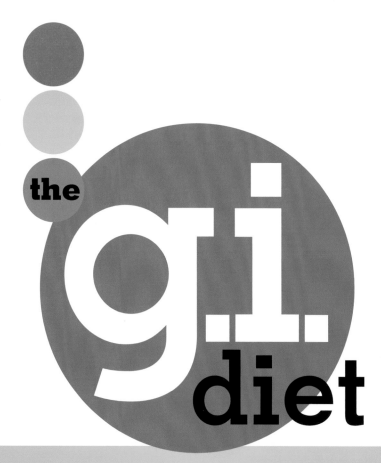

the g.i. diet

THE GREEN-LIGHT WAY
TO PERMANENT WEIGHT LOSS

Revised and Updated

RICK GALLOP

Past President of the Heart and Stroke Foundation of Ontario

Random House Canada

PUBLISHED BY RANDOM HOUSE CANADA

Copyright © 2011 Green Light Foods Inc.

www.randomhouse.ca

Random House Canada and colophon are registered trademarks.

Library and Archives Canada Cataloguing in Publication

Gallop, Rick
    The G.I. diet, 10th anniversary / Rick Gallop.—10th anniversary ed.

Includes index.
Also issued in electronic format.

ISBN 978-0-307-36153-0

    1. Glycemic index. 2. Reducing diets. 3. Reducing diets—Recipes.
I. Title.

RM222.2.G34 2011   613.2'5   C2011-906074-4

Printed and bound in Canada

10 9 8 7 6 5 4 3 2

Contents

Introduction

Since the original G.I. Diet was published ten years ago, over two million copies have been sold in twenty-three countries and seventeen languages, making it the most successful diet and health book in Canadian publishing history.

Perhaps our biggest surprise was both the quantity and quality of feedback from our readers—some 70,000 e-mails! While most of the e-mails talked about how successful the G.I. Diet has been for them, it has become increasingly clear that long-term success depends a great deal on people's ability or willingness to change eating behaviours and lifestyle. The most common refrain was "Please don't call this a diet; it's a lifestyle change."

What also has become apparent is the importance of how personality traits can influence people's approach to food and their long-term success in making a permanent change to a healthy eating lifestyle.

A simple example: Think about how you approach a buffet: do you plunge in and overload your plate without a second thought? Or do you think, "I'll make up for it tomorrow?" Perhaps you think it doesn't matter: "No matter what I do, I'll fail," or you analyze the buffet table then carefully select minute, carefully calculated samples, worrying that you have the precise correct amount? Each of these approaches to that buffet suggests specific personality traits.

Whether you are impulsive, wishful, helpless or controlling, there is little you can do to change your personality. However, this book will help you identify your specific personality traits, examine how they contribute to eating behaviours, and outline how you can use this knowledge to your advantage and modify the potentially negative influences of these characteristics.

The original G.I. Diet promised that you wouldn't go hungry or feel deprived; it is a plan that is simple, not time consuming, and promotes wellness and boosting energy levels. The new, revised G.I. Diet couples all these benefits with a personality-driven guide to changing food behaviours to help make permanent weight loss even easier.

Please visit our website WWW.GIDIET.COM for the latest updates and details of all the other books in the G.I. Diet series including:

- *The G.I. Diet Cookbook* with over 200 delicious green-light recipes.
- *The G.I. Diet Guide to Shopping and Eating Out,* which conveniently fits into pocket or purse.
- *The G.I. Diet Express* for busy people .
- a series of books based on e-clinics we conducted: The *G.I.Diet Clinic* (directed at "big people"), The *G.I. Diet Menopause Clinic* and the *G.I. Diet Diabetes Clinic.*

You may also contact us through our website; we very much look forward to receiving your comments or suggestions.

RICK AND RUTH GALLOP

HOW TO USE THIS BOOK

The first few chapters of the book introduce the principles of the G.I. Diet and explains how it works. You will learn how much weight you should lose and what you can eat, how much and when.

The rest of the book shows you how to put the G.I. Diet into practice. It will help you prepare delicious meals and snacks at home and guide you in making the right choices when dining out. In addition, we've given you the tools to enable you to determine your own personality characteristics and discover how this will help change your eating behaviours and habits that are essential for permanent weight loss.

Chapter One
The Problem

While I was waging my personal battle of the bulge, I couldn't help but be struck by the number of people who were engaged in the same struggle. The statistics are truly astonishing: over 60 percent of Canadian adults today are overweight. That's more than double what it was only ten years ago. Even more worrying is the tripling of the obesity rate among children over the past twenty years. What's happened to us? Why have we gained so much weight in recent years?

The simple explanation is that people are eating too many calories. Unless one denies the basic laws of thermodynamics, the equation never changes: consume more calories than you expend and the surplus is stored in the body as fat. That's the inescapable fact. But that doesn't explain why people today are eating more calories than they used to. To answer that question we must first understand the three key components of any diet—carbohydrates, fats and proteins—and how they work in our digestive system. Since fats are probably the least understood part, let's start with them.

FATS

Fat is definitely a bad word these days, and it engenders an enormous amount of confusion and contradiction. But are you aware that fats are absolutely essential for a nutritious diet? They contain various key elements that are crucial to the digestive process.

The next fact might also surprise you: fat does not necessarily make you fat. The quantity you consume does. And that's something that's often difficult to control, because your body loves fat. Non-fat foods require lots of processing to be transformed into those fat cells around your waist and hips; fatty foods just slide right in. Processing takes energy, and your body hates wasting energy. It needs to expend about 20 to 25 percent of the energy it gets from a non-fat food just to process it. So your body definitely prefers fat, and as we all know from personal experience, it will do everything it can to persuade us to eat more of it. That's why fatty foods like juicy steaks, chocolate and decadent ice creams taste so good to us. But because fat contains twice as many calories per gram as carbohydrates and proteins, we really have to be careful about the amount of fat we eat.

In addition to limiting how much fat we consume, we must also pay attention to the type of fat. While the type of fat has no effect on our weight, it is critical to our health—especially heart health.

There are four types of fat: the best, the better, the bad and the really ugly. The "bad" fats are called saturated fats, and they are easily recognizable because they almost always come from animal sources and they solidify at room temperature. Butter, cheese and meat are all high in saturated fats. There are a couple of others you should be aware of too: coconut oil and palm oil are two vegetable oils that are saturated, and because they are cheap, they are used in many snack foods, especially cookies. Saturated fats are a principal cause of heart disease because they boost cholesterol, which in turn thickens arteries and causes heart attack and stroke. And recent research has demonstrated that several cancers—breast, colon and prostate—as well as Alzheimer's are associated with diets high in saturated fat.

Check your labels.

The "really ugly" fats are potentially the most dangerous. They are vegetable oils that have been heat-treated to make them thicken. These hydrogenated oils take on the worst characteristics of saturated fats, so don't use them, and avoid snack foods, baked goods and cereals that contain them. Check the label for "hydrogenated oils," "partially hydrogenated oils" or "trans fat."

The "better" fats are called polyunsaturated, and they are cholesterol free. Most vegetable oils, such as corn and sunflower, fall into this category. What you should really be using, however, are monounsaturated fats, the "best," which are found in olives, peanuts, almonds, and olive and canola oils. Monounsaturated fats have a beneficial effect on cholesterol and are good for your heart. (See chapter 13 for more information on cholesterol and heart disease.) Though fancy olive oils are expensive, you can get the same health benefits from reasonably priced house brands at your supermarket. Olive oil is used extensively in the famed Mediterranean diet, which is also rich in fruits and vegetables. Because of their diet, southern Europeans have some of the lowest rates of heart disease in the world, and obesity is not a problem in those countries. So look for monounsaturated fats and oils on food labels. Most manufacturers who use them will say so, because they know it's a key selling point for informed consumers.

COOKING OILS/FATS

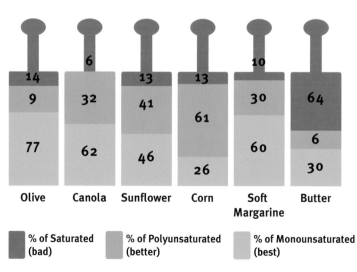

	Olive	Canola	Sunflower	Corn	Soft Margarine	Butter
	14	6	13	13	10	
	9	32	41	61	30	64
	77	62	46	26	60	6
						30

■ % of Saturated (bad)   ■ % of Polyunsaturated (better)   ■ % of Monounsaturated (best)

Another highly beneficial oil, which is in a category of its own, contains a wonderful ingredient called omega-3. This oil is found in deep-sea fish such as salmon and in flax and canola seed. It's extremely good for your heart health (see page 176).

So we know that it's important to avoid the bad and the really ugly fats and to incorporate the best fats in our diets to make our hearts healthy. Many of us have tried to lower our fat intake by using leaner cuts of meat and drinking lower-fat milk. But even with these modifications our fat consumption hasn't decreased. Why? Because many of our favourite foods—like crackers, muffins, cereals and fast foods—contain hidden fats. Detecting them often seems to require an advanced degree in nutrition.

So we're not eating less fat, but contrary to popular belief, neither are we eating more. Fat consumption in this country has remained virtually constant over the past ten years, while obesity numbers have doubled. Obviously, fat isn't the culprit. What has increased is our consumption of grain. Grain is a carbohydrate, so let's look at how carbohydrates work.

CARBOHYDRATES

Unfortunately there is a great deal of misinformation in the marketplace about carbohydrates. Much of it stems from the recent low-carb diet fad, which would have you believe that if you stick to low-carb foods, you'll lose weight. If only it were that simple. The reality is that you need carbs for a healthy diet and you shouldn't avoid them. The key is to choose the right, or good, carbs, like fruit, vegetables, legumes, whole grains, nuts and low-fat dairy products. These foods are the primary source of energy for your body, which converts them into glucose. The glucose dissolves in your bloodstream and is diverted to those parts of your body that use energy, like your muscles and your brain. (It may surprise you to know that when you are resting, your brain uses about two-thirds of the glucose in your system!)

Carbohydrates, therefore, are essential for your body to function. They are rich in fibre, vitamins and minerals, including antioxidants, which we now believe play a critical role in protecting against disease, especially heart disease and cancer. For years we've been advised by doctors, nutritionists and government to eat a low-fat, high-carbohydrate diet. Unfortunately, the most popular carbohydrates are grain based. Just look at the amount of space dedicated to grain-based products in our supermarkets today: huge cracker, cookie and snack-food sections; whole aisles of cereals; numerous shelves of pastas and noodles; and baskets and baskets of bagels, rolls, muffins and loaves of bread. I can remember when bagels were exclusive to the Jewish community; now most food stores carry half a dozen different varieties, and chains of bagel stores are spread across the country. Muffins were never as abundant as they are today.

Another modern food sensation has been pasta, once viewed as an ethnic specialty in North America. That's hard to believe today, with pasta a staple on most restaurant menus and every family's shopping list. Eighty percent of Canadian homes now serve pasta at least once a week. And our snack-food options have multiplied: crackers, tortilla chips, corn chips, pretzels and countless varieties of cookies, to name just a few.

In 1970 the average North American ate about 135 pounds of grain. By 2000 that figure had risen to about 200 pounds. That's a 50 percent increase! Why should we be concerned about this? Aren't wheat, corn and rice low-fat? How could grain be making us fat?

The answer lies in the type of grain we're eating today, most of which is in the form of white flour. White flour starts off as whole wheat. At the mill the whole wheat is steamed and scarified by tiny razor-sharp blades to remove the bran, or outer shell, and the endosperm, the next layer. Then the wheat germ and oil are removed because they turn rancid too quickly to be considered commercially viable. What's left after all that

GRAIN CONSUMPTION (pounds per capita)

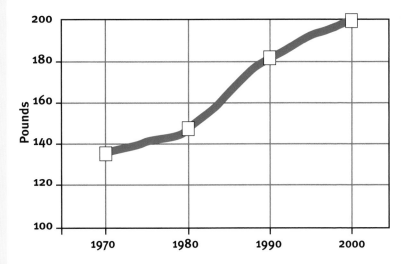

Source: U.S. Department of Agriculture (1970–2000)

processing is unbleached flour, which is then whitened and used to make almost all the breads, bagels, muffins, cookies, crackers, cereals and pastas we consume. Even many "brown" breads are simply artificially coloured white bread.

It's not just grain that's highly processed nowadays. A hundred years ago most of the food people ate came straight from the farm to the dinner table. Lack of refrigeration and scant knowledge of food chemistry meant that most food remained in its original state. However, advances in science, along with the migration of many women out of the kitchen and into the workforce, led to a revolution in prepared foods. Everything became geared to speed and simplicity of preparation. Today's high-speed flour mills use steel rollers rather than the traditional grinding stones to produce an extraordinarily finely ground product, ideal for producing light and fluffy breads and pastries. We now have instant rice and potatoes, as well as entire meals that are ready to eat after just a few minutes in the microwave.

The problem with all this is that the more a food is processed beyond its natural state, the less processing your body has to do to digest it. And the quicker you digest your food, the sooner you are hungry again, and the more you tend to eat. We all know the difference between eating a bowl of old-fashioned slow-cooking oatmeal and a bowl of sugary cold cereal. The oatmeal stays with you—it "sticks to your ribs" as my mother used to say—whereas you are looking for your next meal an hour after eating the bowl of sugary cereal. That's why our ancestors did not have the obesity problem we have today; their foods were basically unprocessed and natural. All the great food companies, like Kraft, General Foods, Kellogg's, McCain, Nabisco and Del Monte, started processing and packaging natural foods only in the past century or so.

Our fundamental problem, then, is that we are eating foods that are too easily digested by our bodies. Clearly, we can't wind back the clock to simpler times, but we need somehow to slow down the digestive process so we feel hungry less often. How can we do that? Well, we have to eat foods that are "slow-release," that break down at a slow and steady rate in our digestive system, leaving us feeling fuller for longer.

How do we identify those "slow-release" foods?

The principal tool to identifying slow-release foods is the glycemic index, which I will now explain. It is the core of this diet and the key to successful weight management.

THE GLYCEMIC INDEX

The glycemic index measures the speed at which you digest food and convert it to glucose, your body's energy source. The faster the food breaks down, the higher the rating on the index. The index sets sugar (glucose) at 100 and scores all foods against that number. Here are some examples:

Baguette	95	Donut	76	Muffin (bran)	56	Oatmeal	42	Fettuccine	32
Instant Rice	87	Cheerios	75	Popcorn low-fat	55	Spaghetti	41	Beans	31
Baked Potatoes	84	Bagel	72	Orange	44	Apple	38	Grapefruit	25
Cornflakes	84	Raisins	64	All-Bran	43	Tomato	38	Fat- and sugar-free Yogurt	14

The chart on the next page illustrates the impact of sugar on the level of glucose in your bloodstream compared with kidney beans, which have a low G.I. rating. As you can see, there is a dramatic difference between the two. Sugar is quickly converted into glucose, which dissolves in your bloodstream, spiking its glucose level. It also disappears quickly, leaving you wanting more. Have you ever eaten a large Chinese meal, with lots of noodles and rice, only to find yourself hungry again an hour or two later? That's because your body rapidly converted the rice and noodles, high-G.I. foods, to glucose, which then quickly disappeared from your bloodstream. Something most of us experience regularly is the feeling of lethargy that follows an hour or so after a fast-food lunch, which generally consists of high-G.I. foods. The surge of glucose followed by the rapid drain leaves us starved of energy. So what do we do? Around mid-afternoon we look for a quick sugar fix, or snack, to bring us out of the slump. A few cookies or a bag of chips cause another rush of glucose, which disappears a short time later—and so the vicious cycle continues. No wonder we're a nation of snackers!

When you eat a high-G.I. food and experience a rapid spike in blood sugar, your pancreas releases the hormone insulin. Insulin does two things extremely well. First, it reduces the level of glucose in your bloodstream by diverting it into various body tissues for immediate short-term use or by storing it as fat—which is why glucose disappears so quickly.

G.I. IMPACT ON SUGAR LEVELS

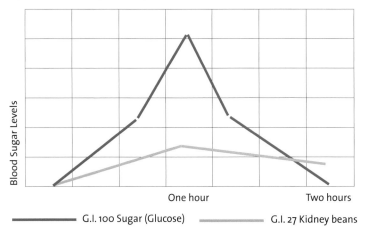

Blood Sugar Levels

One hour   Two hours

——— G.I. 100 Sugar (Glucose)   ——— G.I. 27 Kidney beans

Second, it inhibits the conversion of body fat back into glucose for the body to burn. This evolutionary feature is a throwback to the days when our ancestors were hunter-gatherers, habitually experiencing times of feast or famine. When food was in abundance, the body stored its surplus as fat to tide it over the inevitable days of famine. Insulin was the champion in this process, both helping to accumulate fat and then guarding its depletion.

Today, everything has changed except our stomachs. A digestive system that has taken millions of years to evolve is, in a comparative evolutionary blink of an eye, expected to cope with a food revolution. We don't have to hunt and search for food any more; we have a guaranteed supply of highly processed foods with a multitude of tempting flavours and textures at the supermarket. Not only are we consuming more easily digested calories, but we're not expending as much energy in finding our food and keeping ourselves warm—the two major preoccupations of our ancestors.

Since insulin is the key trigger to storing glucose as well as the sentry that keeps those fat cells intact, it is crucial to maintain low insulin levels when you are trying to lose weight, and that means avoiding high-G.I. foods. Low-G.I. foods such as apples are like the tortoise to the high-G.I. foods' hare. They break down in your digestive system at a slow, steady rate. You don't get a quick sugar fix when you eat them, but, tortoiselike, they stay the course, so that you feel full longer. Therefore if you want to lose weight, you must stick to low-G.I. foods.

But the fact that a food has a low G.I. does not necessarily make it desirable. The other critical factor determining whether a food will allow us to lose weight is its calorie content. It's the combination of low-G.I foods with fewer calories, i.e., low in sugar and fat, that is the "magic bullet" of the G.I. Diet. Low-G.I., low-calorie foods make you feel more satiated than do foods with a high G.I. and calorie level. Later in this book I will provide you with a comprehensive chart identifying the foods that will make you fat and those that will allow you to lose weight. Don't expect the low-G.I. foods to be tasteless and boring! There are many delicious and satisfying choices that will make you feel as though you aren't even on a diet.

There are three other important components that inhibit the rapid breakdown of food in our digestive system: fibre, fat and protein.

Fibre, in simple terms, provides low-calorie filler. It does double duty, in fact: it literally fills up your stomach, so you feel satiated, and your body takes much longer to break it down, so it stays with you longer and slows the digestive process. There are two forms of fibre: soluble and insoluble. Soluble fibre is found in foods such as oatmeal, beans, barley and citrus fruits, and has been shown to lower blood cholesterol levels. Insoluble fibre is important for normal bowel function and is typically found in whole wheat breads and cereals, and most vegetables.

Fat, like fibre, acts as a brake in the digestive process. When combined with other foods it becomes a barrier to digestive juices. It also signals the brain that you are satisfied and do not require more food. But we know that many fats are harmful to your heart, and they contain twice the number of calories per gram as carbohydrates and protein. Since protein also acts as a brake in the digestive process, let's look at it in more detail.

PROTEIN

One-half of your dry body weight is made up of protein, i.e., your muscles, organs, skin and hair. Obviously protein is an essential part of your diet. It's required to build and repair body tissue, and figures in nearly all metabolic reactions.

Protein is also much more effective than carbohydrates or fat in satisfying hunger. It will make you feel fuller longer, which is why you should always try to incorporate some protein in every meal and snack. It will help keep you alert and feeling full. Again, however, the type of protein you consume is important. Proteins are found in a broad range of food products, both animal and vegetable, and not just in red meat and whole dairy products, which are high in saturated or "bad" fat.

So what sort of protein should you be including in your diet? Choose low-fat proteins: lean or low-fat cuts of meat that have been trimmed of any visible fat; skinless poultry; fresh, frozen or canned fish (but not the kind that's coated with batter, which is invariably high in fat); low-fat dairy products like skim milk (believe it or not, after a couple of weeks of drinking it, it tastes just like 2%); low-fat yogurt (look for the artificially sweetened versions, as many manufacturers pump up the sugar as they drop the fat) and low-fat cottage cheese; liquid eggs or egg whites and tofu. To most people's surprise the best source of protein may well be the humble bean. Beans are high protein, low fat and high fibre, and they break down slowly in your digestive system, so you feel fuller longer. They can also be added to foods like soups and salads to boost their protein and fibre content. Nuts too are a fine source of protein, with a good monounsaturated fat content. However, because they are so high in calories, you must limit the quantity. Perhaps the simplest way to boost your protein intake is flavoured whey isolate protein powder, which comes in large plastic jars and is readily available at your supermarket, health food store or pharmacy. Simply add a tablespoon or two to your breakfast cereal or mix with a glass of skim milk for a delicious protein drink any time of day.

One of the most important things you should know about protein is to spread your daily allowance across all your meals. Too often we grab a hasty breakfast of coffee and toast—a protein-free meal. Lunch is sometimes not much better: a bowl of pasta with steamed vegetables or a green salad with garlic bread. Where's the protein? A typical afternoon snack of a cookie, piece of fruit or muffin contains not a gram of protein. Generally, it's not until dinner that we include protein in our meal, usually our entire daily recommended allowance plus some extra. Because protein is a critical brain food, providing amino acids for the neurotransmitters that relay messages in the brain, it would be better to load up on protein earlier in the day rather than later. That would give you an alert and active mind for your daily activities. However, as I have said, the best solution is to spread your protein consumption throughout the day. This will help keep you on the ball and feeling full.

Now that we know how carbohydrates, fats and proteins work in our digestive system and what makes us gain weight, let's use the science to put together an eating plan that will take off the extra pounds. First, though, let's look at how much weight you should be trying to lose.

Chapter Two
How Much Weight Should I Lose?

In this age of excessively and often unhealthily skinny supermodels and TV stars, it's easy to lose sight of what is a healthy weight. Your skin, bones, organs, hair—everything—contribute to your total weight. The only part that you want to reduce is your excess fat, so that's what we have to determine.

There have been many techniques designed to measure excess fat, from measuring pinches of fat (which can be quite misleading) to convoluted formulas and tables requiring higher math. The best method is the Body Mass Index, or BMI, which is the only internationally accepted measurement for assessing how much fat you are carrying relative to your height. I've included a BMI table on pages 16 to 17 and it's very simple to use.

Just find your height in the top horizontal column and your weight in the left vertical column. Where the two columns intersect is your BMI.

You will have noted that BMI tables have a broad range of weights in each of the weight categories: healthy weight (BMI 19–24), overweight (BMI 25–29) and obese (BMI 30 and over). For instance, a 5'5" woman has a healthy weight range from 114 pounds (BMI 19) to 144 pounds (BMI 24). The reason for this broad range is primarily to allow for variances in people's different frame sizes.

Women with small frames should have a healthy weight in the bottom third of the range while those with large frames should be in the top third; i.e., small frame, BMI 19–21; medium frame, BMI 21–22; large frame, BMI 23–24.

BMI TABLE

WEIGHT (POUNDS) \ HEIGHT (FT INS)	4'6"	4'8"	4'10"	5'0"	5'2"	5'3"	5'4"	5'5"	5'6"	5'7"	5'8"	5'9"	5'10"	5'11"	6'0"	6'2"	6'4"	6'6"	6'8"
91	22.0	20.4	19.0	17.8	16.6	16.1	15.6	15.1	14.7	14.3	13.8	13.4	13.1	12.7	12.3	11.7	11.1	10.5	10.0
94	22.7	21.1	19.6	18.4	17.2	16.7	16.1	15.6	15.2	14.7	14.3	13.9	13.5	13.1	12.7	12.1	11.4	10.9	10.3
98	23.7	22.0	20.5	19.1	17.9	17.4	16.8	16.3	15.8	15.3	14.9	14.5	14.1	13.7	13.3	12.6	11.9	11.3	10.8
101	24.4	22.6	21.1	19.7	18.5	17.9	17.3	16.8	16.3	15.8	15.4	14.9	14.5	14.1	13.7	13.0	12.3	11.7	11.1
105	25.4	23.5	21.9	20.5	19.2	18.6	18.0	17.5	16.9	16.4	16.0	15.5	15.1	14.6	14.2	13.5	12.8	12.1	11.5
108	26.1	24.2	22.6	21.1	19.8	19.1	18.5	18.0	17.4	16.9	16.4	15.9	15.5	15.1	14.6	13.9	13.1	12.5	11.9
112	27.1	25.1	23.4	21.9	20.5	19.8	19.2	18.6	18.1	17.5	17.0	16.5	16.1	15.6	15.2	14.4	13.6	12.9	12.3
115	27.8	25.8	24.0	22.5	21.0	20.4	19.7	19.1	18.6	18.0	17.5	17.0	16.5	16.0	15.6	14.8	14.0	13.3	12.6
119	28.8	26.7	24.9	23.2	21.8	21.1	20.4	19.8	19.2	18.6	18.1	17.6	17.1	16.6	16.1	15.3	14.5	13.8	13.1
122	29.5	27.4	25.5	23.8	22.3	21.6	20.9	20.3	19.7	19.1	18.5	18.0	17.5	17.0	16.5	15.7	14.9	14.1	13.4
129	31.2	28.9	27.0	25.2	23.6	22.9	22.1	21.5	20.8	20.2	19.6	19.0	18.5	18.0	17.5	16.6	15.7	14.9	14.2
133	32.1	29.8	27.8	26.0	24.3	23.6	22.8	22.1	21.5	20.8	20.2	19.6	19.1	18.5	18.0	17.1	16.2	15.4	14.6
136	32.9	30.5	28.4	26.6	24.9	24.1	23.3	22.6	22.0	21.3	20.7	20.1	19.5	19.0	18.4	17.5	16.6	15.7	14.9
140	33.8	31.4	29.3	27.3	25.6	24.8	24.0	23.3	22.6	21.9	21.3	20.7	20.1	19.5	19.0	18.0	17.0	16.2	15.4
143	34.6	32.1	29.9	27.9	26.2	25.3	24.5	23.8	23.1	22.4	21.7	21.1	20.5	19.9	19.4	18.4	17.4	16.5	15.7
147	35.5	33.0	30.7	28.7	26.9	26.0	25.2	24.5	23.7	23.0	22.4	21.7	21.1	20.5	19.9	18.9	17.9	17.0	16.1
150	36.3	33.6	31.3	29.3	27.4	26.6	25.7	25.0	24.2	23.5	22.8	22.2	21.5	20.9	20.3	19.3	18.3	17.3	16.5
154	37.2	34.5	32.2	30.1	28.2	27.3	26.4	25.6	24.9	24.1	23.4	22.7	22.1	21.5	20.9	19.8	18.7	17.8	16.9
157	37.9	35.2	32.8	30.7	28.7	27.8	26.9	26.1	25.3	24.6	23.9	23.2	22.5	21.9	21.3	20.2	19.1	18.1	17.2
161	38.9	36.1	33.6	31.4	29.4	28.5	27.6	26.8	26.0	25.2	24.5	23.8	23.1	22.5	21.8	20.7	19.6	18.6	17.7
164	39.6	36.8	34.3	32.0	30.0	29.1	28.2	27.3	26.5	25.7	24.9	24.2	23.5	22.9	22.2	21.1	20.0	19.0	18.0
168	40.6	37.7	35.1	32.8	30.7	29.8	28.8	28.0	27.1	26.3	25.5	24.8	24.1	23.4	22.8	21.6	20.4	19.4	18.5
171	41.3	38.3	35.7	33.4	31.3	30.3	29.4	28.5	27.6	26.8	26.0	25.3	24.5	23.8	23.2	22.0	20.8	19.8	18.8
175	42.3	39.2	36.6	34.2	32.0	31.0	30.0	29.1	28.2	27.4	26.6	25.8	25.1	24.4	23.7	22.5	21.3	20.2	19.2

BMI RATING	INDICATIONS
19–24	Healthy weight
25–29	Overweight
30–39	Obese
40 plus	Morbidly obese

178	19.6	20.6	21.7	22.9	24.1	24.8	25.5	26.3	27.1	27.9	28.7	29.6	30.6	31.5	32.6	34.8	37.2	39.9	43.0
182	20.0	21.0	22.2	23.4	24.7	25.4	26.1	26.9	27.7	28.5	29.4	30.3	31.2	32.2	33.3	35.5	38.0	40.8	44.0
185	20.3	21.4	22.5	23.8	25.1	25.8	26.5	27.3	28.1	29.0	29.9	30.8	31.8	32.8	33.8	36.1	38.7	41.5	44.7
189	20.8	21.8	23.0	24.3	25.6	26.4	27.1	27.9	28.7	29.6	30.5	31.5	32.4	33.5	34.6	36.9	39.5	42.4	45.7
192	21.1	22.2	23.4	24.7	26.0	26.8	27.5	28.4	29.2	30.1	31.0	31.9	33.0	34.0	35.1	37.5	40.1	43.0	46.4
196	21.5	22.6	23.9	25.2	26.6	27.3	28.1	28.9	29.8	30.7	31.6	32.6	33.6	34.7	35.8	38.3	41.0	43.9	47.4
199	21.9	23.0	24.2	25.5	27.0	27.8	28.6	29.4	30.3	31.2	32.1	33.1	34.2	35.3	36.4	38.9	41.6	44.6	48.1
203	22.3	23.5	24.7	26.1	27.5	28.3	29.1	30.0	30.9	31.8	32.8	33.8	34.8	36.0	37.1	39.6	42.4	45.5	49.1
206	22.6	23.8	25.1	26.4	27.9	28.7	29.6	30.4	31.3	32.3	33.2	34.3	35.4	36.5	37.7	40.2	43.1	46.2	49.8
210	23.1	24.3	25.6	27.0	28.5	29.3	30.1	31.0	31.9	32.9	33.9	34.9	36.0	37.2	38.4	41.0	43.9	47.1	50.8
213	23.4	24.6	25.9	27.3	28.9	29.7	30.6	31.5	32.4	33.4	34.4	35.4	36.6	37.7	39.0	41.6	44.5	47.8	51.5
217	23.8	25.1	26.4	27.9	29.4	30.3	31.1	32.0	33.0	34.0	35.0	36.1	37.2	38.4	39.7	42.4	45.4	48.6	52.4
220	24.2	25.4	26.8	28.2	29.8	30.7	31.6	32.5	33.5	34.5	35.5	36.6	37.8	39.0	40.2	43.0	46.0	49.3	53.2
224	24.6	25.9	27.3	28.8	30.4	31.2	32.1	33.1	34.1	35.1	36.2	37.3	38.4	39.7	41.0	43.7	46.8	50.2	54.1
227	24.9	26.2	27.6	29.1	30.8	31.7	32.6	33.5	34.5	35.6	36.6	37.8	39.0	40.2	41.5	44.3	47.4	50.9	54.9
231	25.4	26.7	28.1	29.7	31.3	32.2	33.1	34.1	35.1	36.2	37.3	38.4	39.7	40.9	42.2	45.1	48.3	51.8	55.8
234	25.7	27.0	28.5	30.0	31.7	32.6	33.6	34.6	35.6	36.6	37.8	38.9	40.2	41.5	42.8	45.7	48.9	52.5	56.6
238	26.1	27.5	29.0	30.6	32.3	33.2	34.1	35.1	36.2	37.3	38.4	39.6	40.9	42.2	43.5	46.5	49.7	53.4	57.5
245	26.9	28.3	29.8	31.4	33.2	34.1	35.1	36.1	37.2	38.3	39.5	40.7	42.0	43.3	44.8	47.8	51.2	54.9	59.0
252	27.6	29.1	30.5	32.3	34.1	35.1	36.1	37.2	38.3	39.4	40.6	41.9	43.2	44.6	46.0	49.2	52.6	56.4	60.7
259	28.4	29.9	31.5	33.2	35.1	36.1	37.1	38.2	39.3	40.5	41.8	43.0	44.4	45.8	47.3	50.5	54.1	58.0	62.4
266	29.2	30.7	32.3	34.1	36.0	37.0	38.1	39.2	40.4	41.6	42.9	44.2	45.6	47.1	48.6	51.9	55.5	59.6	64.1

To calculate your frame, here is a guide for women based on wrist measurement. Take the measurement with a tape measure at the narrowest point on your wrist.

Wrist Size in inches	Height Under 5'2"	Height 5'2"–5'5"	Height Over 5'5"
Under 5.50	S	S	S
5.50–5.75	M	S	S
5.75–6.00	L	S	S
6.00–6.25	L	M	S
6.25–6.50	L	L	M
Over 6.50	L	L	L

Key: S = Small frame; M = Medium frame; L = Large frame.

For males it is a little simpler. All males 5'5" and over, the wrist measurements are simply:
Wrist measurement under 6.5 inches = small frame
Wrist measurement of 6.5–7 .5 inches = medium frame
Wrist measurement over 7.5 inches = large frame
Source: U.S. National Library of Medicine

If you are over 65 years, I suggest you allow yourself an extra 10 pounds to help protect you in case of a fall or long illness. Basically everyone has their own particular body makeup, metabolism and genes, so there are no hard-and-fast rules for exactly how much you should weigh. The BMI table is a guide, not an absolute.

However, it is important to **set your goals**. Everyone has different motivations for losing weight and neither I nor the BMI tables can do this for you. So set your target-weight goals and write them down.

Remember, you are starting on a journey. Don't expect miracles. The weight will come off.

For those with a BMI of over 30 who may feel overwhelmed by the task ahead, you do have one advantage over your skinnier compatriots in that you will lose weight at a faster rate.

Say you've decided to target a BMI of 22. Put your finger on your height and run it down until you reach the BMI number 22 (or a fraction close enough). Then run your finger across to the number (in pounds) across the bottom. This is what your weight should be to achieve your BMI target. Let's look at an example: Mary is 5 feet 6 inches and weighs 178 pounds. Her current BMI is 28.7, but she'd like to have a BMI of 22. This means Mary has to lose 42 pounds in order to bring her to her 22 BMI goal of 136 pounds.

Another measurement that is important to know is your waist circumference. This measurement is an even better indication of your health than your weight is. Recent research has shown that abdominal fat acts almost like a separate organ in the body—only this "organ" is a destructive one. It releases harmful proteins and free fatty acids, increasing the risk of heart disease, stroke, cancer and diabetes. Thus women with a waist circumference of 35 inches or more and men with 37 inches or more are at risk of endangering their health. And women with a waist circumference of 37 inches or more and men with 40 inches or more are at serious risk of heart disease, stroke, cancer and diabetes. Doctors describe people with abdominal fat as apple shaped.

To measure your waist, take a measuring tape and wrap it around your natural waist just above the navel. Don't be tempted to do a walk-down-the-beach-and-suck-it-in routine. Just stand in a relaxed position and keep the measuring tape from cutting into your flesh.

The 42 pounds that Mary has to lose are pounds of fat—Mary's energy storage tank. In order for her to lose weight she must access and draw down those fat cells. This reminds me of a peculiar contraption used in England during the Second World War. The famous double-decker buses had their upper deck converted into a natural gas tank, consisting of a large fabric balloon. When full, the balloon puffed up several feet above the top of the bus. As it proceeded along its route, the balloon slowly deflated, disappearing by the end of its destination, where it was re-inflated. That's how I visualize our body fat: a deflating balloon from which we draw down our energy, except that in our case the balloon is around our waist, hips and thighs!

So how do you draw down energy from your fat cells? By consuming fewer calories than your body needs. This will force your body to start using its fat stores to make up for the shortfall. Now, I know no one wants to hear about calories, particularly those of us who've tried long and hard to lose weight. Nevertheless, unless you are among those rare and blessed people whose metabolism and genetics enable them to eat as much as they want without gaining an ounce—and if you are, why would you be reading this book?—you, like me and the rest of us mere mortals, are doomed to the inevitable equation. But don't be disheartened: you can easily reduce your daily calorie intake without going hungry and without having to calculate the number of calories in everything you put in your mouth.

I promised you a simple eating plan that reflects the real world we live in, and that is what I'll give you. The plan is divided into two phases. In Phase I you'll be reducing your caloric intake, burning off those excess fat cells and slimming down to a healthy, ideal weight. This phase takes between three and six months, and it's really a matter of simple math. A pound of fat contains around 3,600 calories. To lose that pound in one week you must reduce your caloric intake by around 500 calories per day (500 × 7 days = 3,500 calories). So if you want to lose twenty pounds, it will take approximately twenty weeks.

But this formula is for people who have to lose about 10 percent of their body weight. If you have more to lose, the good news is that you will in all likelihood drop more pounds per week. The higher your BMI, the faster you will lose weight. People with a BMI of 30 and over frequently lose an average of 2 to 3 pounds per week.

Talking of scales, it is important that you are able to have an accurate measure of your weight. Many of you are probably using scales you have had around for years, and they are likely the analogue type (either with a pointer or a rotating disk). Over time, the springs stretch and the scale will become wildly inaccurate. Do yourself a favour and purchase an inexpensive digital scale.

If twenty weeks seems like a long time to be on a diet, think of it in terms of the rest of your life. What's half a year compared with the many, many years you'll spend afterward with a slim, healthy body? This isn't a fad diet—fad diets don't work. In fact, the sole reason that 95 percent of diets don't lead to permanent weight loss is simply that people can't or won't stay on them. And the reasons are very simple: people feel hungry or deprived; they get tired of counting calories, points or carbs; or they feel lethargic and depressed.

With the G.I. Diet, however, you will not feel hungry or deprived; you'll never have to count calories or points again, and you will rediscover energy levels you thought you had lost forever.

The most important message I can give you is that if you wish to permanently lose weight, you have to permanently change the way you eat. The most common single theme I hear from successful G.I. Diet readers is that this is not so much a diet as a new and permanent way of eating. The G.I. Diet is a wholesome and surefire route to permanent weight loss.

The reason I've included all this math is to help you

understand this diet and how it's going to work for you. But I don't want you to think that you're going to have to do any calculations yourself! They're all built into the program. I've done all the math, calculations and measurements for you, and sorted the foods you like to eat into one of three categories based on the colours of a traffic light. This easy-to-follow colour-coded system means you will never have to count calories or points ever again.

When you've reached your target BMI, Phase II begins. Here, your calorie input and output are balanced. You're no longer trying to lose weight, so we have relaxed the rules a little. This is how you'll be eating the rest of your life. Sound simple? It is! So let's get going with Phase I.

Chapter Three
Phase I

With the theory and science of the G.I. Diet behind us, it's time to get practical! As you know, Phase I is the weight-loss portion of the program, so let's get into the details: what to eat, how much and how often.

WHAT DO I EAT?
To find out what to eat and what to avoid, check out the Complete G.I. Diet Food Guide on pages 183–192.

Here's how the colour-coded categories work:

RED-LIGHT FOODS
The foods in the red column are to be avoided. They are high G.I., higher-calorie foods, and frequently have high saturated fat levels.

YELLOW-LIGHT FOODS
The foods in the yellow column are mid-range G.I. foods and should be treated with caution. There are two phases in the G.I. Diet: Phase I is the weight-loss portion of the diet and yellow-light foods should be avoided during this time. Once you've reached your target weight, you enter Phase II, the maintenance phase, and you can begin to enjoy yellow-light foods from time to time.

GREEN-LIGHT FOODS
The green column lists foods that are low G.I., low in saturated fat and lower in calories. These are the foods that will help you lose weight. Don't expect them to be tasteless and boring! The many delicious and satisfying choices will make you feel as though you aren't even on a diet

You might be surprised to find potatoes and rice in the green-light column, but they are fine as long as they are the right type. Baked potatoes and french fries have a high G.I., while boiled small (preferably new) potatoes have a lower G.I. Short-grain glutinous (sticky) rice served in Chinese and Thai restaurants is high G.I., while long-grain, brown, basmati and wild rice are low G.I. Pasta is also a green-light food—as long as it is cooked only until *al dente* (with some firmness to the bite). Any processing of food, including cooking, increases its G.I. since heat breaks down food starch capsules and fibre, giving your digestive juices a head start. This is why you should never overcook vegetables; instead microwave or steam them until they are tender. This way they will retain their vitamins and other nutrients, and their G.I. rating will remain low. Remember, the objective is to have foods digest slowly; avoid anything that increases the speed of digestion such as raising the G.I. level of foods.

In the next chapter, we will outline the best green-light options for breakfast, lunch, dinner and snacks.

HOW MUCH DO I EAT?

The G.I. Diet calls for three meals and three snacks daily. My mother liked to say that the devil finds work for idle hands. Your stomach works on a similar principle in that if it's not kept busy processing food and steadily supplying energy to your brain and muscles, it will be looking for its next meal!

With a few exceptions that I outline below, you can eat as much of the green-light foods as you like. However, this does call for some common sense and moderation. Three oranges or two heads of cabbage at a sitting is not moderation!

GREEN-LIGHT SERVING SIZES

Crispbreads (with high fibre, e.g., Wasa Fibre)	2 crispbreads
Green-light breads (which have at least 3 grams of fibre per slice)	1 slice
Green-light cereals	1/2 cup
Green-light nuts	8 to 10
Margarine (non-hydrogenated, light)	2 teaspoons
Meat, fish, poultry	4 ounces (about the size of a pack of cards)
Olive/canola oil	1 teaspoon
Olives	4 to 5
Pasta	1 cup cooked
Potatoes (boiled, preferably new)	2 to 3
Rice (basmati, brown, long grain)	2/3 cup cooked

PORTIONS

Each meal and snack should contain, if possible, a combination of green-light protein, carbohydrates—especially fruit and vegetables—and fats. An easy way to visualize portion size is to divide your plate into three sections (see illustration on p. 26). Half the plate should be filled with at least two vegetables; one-quarter should contain protein, such as lean meat, poultry, seafood, eggs or tofu; and the last quarter should contain a green-light serving of rice, pasta or potatoes.

One of the simplest ways to reduce your portion sizes is to change your huge dinner plates to luncheon-size plates. Research has shown that this is a highly effective way of reducing caloric intake without creating a feeling of being shortchanged.

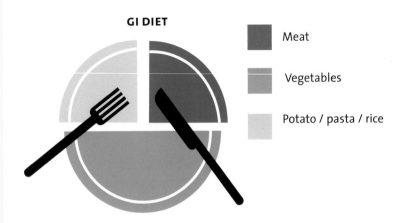

GI DIET

- Meat
- Vegetables
- Potato / pasta / rice

WHEN DO I EAT?

Try to eat regularly throughout the day. If you skimp on breakfast and lunch you will probably be starving by dinner and end up overeating. Have one snack mid-morning, another mid-afternoon and one before bed. The idea is to keep your digestive system happily busy so you won't start craving those red-light snacks.

Chapter 4
Meal Basics

So what can you eat? Let's talk about breakfast first.

BREAKFAST

I know you've been told that breakfast is the most important meal of the day, and it's actually true. It's the first thing you eat following your night-long "fast" of twelve hours or more, and it launches you into your workday. Eating a healthy breakfast will help you avoid the need to grab a coffee and pastry as soon as you hit the office, and it will make you feel satisfied and energetic. Eating breakfast every day doesn't mean you have to set the alarm any earlier. If you have time to read the paper or feed the cat, you have time to prepare and eat a green-light breakfast.

The following chart lists typical breakfast foods in the colour-coded categories. For a full list of foods, see the Complete G.I. Diet Food Guide on pages 183–92.

BREAKFAST	RED	YELLOW	GREEN
PROTEIN			
Meat and Eggs	Regular bacon	Turkey bacon	Back bacon
	Sausages	Whole regular eggs (preferably omega-3)	Lean ham
			Liquid eggs/egg whites
Dairy	Cheese	Cream cheese (light)	Buttermilk
	Cottage cheese (whole or 2%)	Milk (1%)	Cottage/cream cheese or sour cream (1% or fat-free)

BREAKFAST	RED	YELLOW	GREEN
	Cream	Sour cream (light)	Extra-low-fat cheese
	Milk (whole or 2%)	Yogurt (low-fat with sugar)	Fruit yogurt (fat-free with sweetener)
	Sour cream		Milk (skim)
	Yogurt (whole or 2%)		Soy milk (plain, low-fat)
CARBOHYDRATES			
Cereals	All cold cereals except those listed as yellow- or green-light	Kashi Good Friends	All-Bran
	Granola	Shredded Wheat Bran	Bran Buds
	Muesli (commercial)		Fibre First
			Kashi Go Lean
			Kashi Go Lean Crunch
			Oat Bran
			Porridge (large flake or steel cut)
			Red River
Breads/ Grains	Bagels	Crispbreads (with fibre)*	Crispbreads (high fibre, e.g., Wasa Fibre)*
	Baguette	Whole-grain breads*	Green-light muffins (see pp. 108-10)
	Cookies		Whole-grain, high-fibre breads (min. 3 g fibre per slice)*
	Doughnuts		
	Muffins		
	Pancakes/Waffles		
	White bread		
Fruits (Fresh/ Frozen)	Applesauce containing sugar	Apricots (fresh and dried)**	Apples
	Canned fruit in syrup	Bananas	Berries
	Melons	Fruit cocktail in juice	Cherries

BREAKFAST	RED	YELLOW	GREEN
	Most dried fruit	Kiwi	Grapefruit
		Mango	Grapes
		Papaya	Oranges
		Pineapple	Peaches
Juices	Fruit drinks	Apple (unsweetened)	Eat the fruit rather than drink its juice
	Prune	Grapefruit (unsweetened)	
	Sweetened juices	Orange (unsweetened)	
	Watermelon	Pear (unsweetened)	
Vege-tables	French fries		Most vegetables
	Hash browns		
FATS			
	Butter	Most nuts	Almonds*
	Hard margarine	Natural nut butters	Canola oil*
	Peanut butter (regular and light)	Peanut butter (100% peanuts)	Hazelnuts*
	Tropical oils	Peanut oil	Olive oil*
	Vegetable shortening	Soft margarine (non-hydrogenated)	Soft margarine (non-hydrogenated, light)*
		Vegetable oils	

* Limit serving size (see page 25).
** For baking, it is acceptable to use a modest amount of dried apricots or cranberries.

Let's take a closer look at some of the usual breakfast choices.

JUICE

● Always eat the fruit or vegetable, rather than drink its juice. The fruit contains more nutrients and fibre than its juice does. This is particularly true of commercially prepared juices. Also, because juice is a processed product, it is more rapidly digested than the parent fruit. To illustrate the point: diabetics who run into an insulin crisis and are in a state of hypoglycemia (low blood sugar) are usually given orange juice, which is a fast way to get glucose into the bloodstream. This is exactly the reverse of what we are trying to achieve. Even worse, a glass of juice has 2.5 times the calories of a fresh whole orange.

CEREALS

- Large-flake or slow-cooking porridge oats are the best choice for two reasons: oatmeal stays with you all morning, and it's great for your heart as it lowers cholesterol. (The cooking time is only around three minutes in the microwave.) Oatmeal is my favourite breakfast. I add fat-free fruit yogurt, sliced almonds and some berries. Delicious!
- Among cold cereals, go for the high-fibre products—the ones that have at least 10 grams of fibre per serving. Fibre content is clearly indicated on cereal packages. Though these cereals are not lots of fun in themselves, you can liven them up by adding fresh or frozen fruits, berries and nuts. There are also one or two high-protein cereals (e.g., Kashi Go Lean), which are a good green-light choice. Look for a minimum of 10 grams of protein per serving.

DAIRY

- The beverage of choice is skim milk. I had a real problem with skim milk both on cereal and as a beverage, but I persevered. Move down from 2% to 1% to skim in stages. I find that 2% tastes like cream now!
- Yogurt is a real plus. But look for low- or no-fat versions with sugar substitute rather than sugar. Regular low-fat yogurts have nearly twice the calories as the versions with sweetener. (There has been a considerable amount of negative publicity and misinformation, generated principally by the sugar industry, about sugar substitutes. This has triggered dozens of studies worldwide, none of which have shown any long-term risks to our health. These products are safe and of real value in calorie control.

But, as with most foods, don't go overboard. Our family favourite is Splenda, which unlike aspartame, can also be used in baking.)

- Your best choice is non-fat Greek-style yogurt. It contains three to four times the protein content of other yogurts even though it's a little more expensive and sometimes difficult to find. (Tip: President's Choice has recently launched an excellent version that is readily available.)
- Cottage cheese is an excellent and filling source of protein. Again, go for the 1% or fat-free variety. Add fruit or light fruit spreads for flavour.
- Use other dairy products sparingly. Avoid most cheeses like the plague; their high saturated fat heads straight for your arteries. The dairy industry has a lot to answer for when it comes to our health. The success of their massive cheese advertising and promotion campaigns, often aimed at children, is reprehensible. If cheese is your thing, then go for the no-fat options or use stronger-flavoured ones, such as Stilton or feta, sprinkled sparingly as a flavour enhancer.

BREAD
- Always use 100 percent whole wheat, or any other whole-grain bread that has a minimum of 3 grams of fibre per slice. Limit yourself to one slice per meal.

EGGS
- Choose low-cholesterol, low-fat eggs in liquid form such as Nutraegg Break Free or Omega Pro (250 mL carton = 5 eggs). Unlike regular eggs, which are high in cholesterol, eggs in liquid form are a great green-light product. Go for them.

SPREADS
- Do not use butter. The latest premium brands of light non-hydrogenated soft margarine are acceptable, but use sparingly.

- Avoid all fruit spreads where the first ingredient is sugar. Look for the "double fruit no added sugar" versions. These taste terrific, are more nutritious and are remarkably low in calories. They are wonderful flavour boosters for oatmeal, high-fibre cereal and cottage cheese.

BACON
- Sorry, but regular bacon is a red-light food. Acceptable alternatives are Canadian back bacon, turkey bacon and lean ham.

COFFEE
- Coffee ideally should be decaffeinated because caffeine stimulates appetite. You can also try switching to tea, which contains significantly less caffeine than coffee . However, if you can't face a day without your morning jolt of java, then go for it, but make sure you have only one cup per day. Never add sugar and use only 1% or skim milk.

For more breakfast suggestions and recipes see chapter 8.

LUNCH

Because lunch is the meal most of us eat outside the home, it can be the most problematic, limited by time, budget and availability considerations. However, with a little strategizing you'll have no problem eating the green-light way. You have two options: brown-bag your lunch, packing items from your green-light pantry, or eat out at a restaurant or fast-food outlet. For a list of foods see the Complete G.I. Diet Food Guide on pages 183–92.

LUNCH	RED	YELLOW	GREEN
PROTEIN			
Meat, Poultry, Fish, Eggs and Meat Substitutes	Ground beef (more than 10% fat)	Ground beef (lean)	All fish and seafood, fresh, frozen (no batter or breading) or canned (in water)
	Hamburgers	Lamb (lean cuts)	Beef (lean cuts)
	Hot dogs	Pork (lean cuts)	Chicken/Turkey breast (skinless)
	Pâté	Tofu (firm)	Egg whites
	Processed meats	Turkey bacon	Ground beef (extra-lean)
	Regular bacon	Whole regular eggs (preferably omega-3)	Lean deli meats
	Sausages	Chicken/turkey leg (skinless)	Liquid eggs (e.g., Break Free)
			Tofu (soft)
			Veal
CARBOHYDRATES			
Breads/Grains	Bagels	Crispbreads (with fibre, e.g., Ryvita High Fibre)	Crispbreads (high fibre, e.g., Wasa Fibre)*
	Baguette/Croissants	Pita (whole wheat)	Pasta (fettuccine, spaghetti, penne, vermicelli, linguine, macaroni)*
	Croutons	Tortillas (whole wheat)	Pita (high fibre)
	Cake/Cookies	Whole-grain breads*	Quinoa
	Hamburger/Hot dog buns		Rice (basmati, wild, brown, long-grain)*
	Macaroni and cheese		Whole-grain, high-fibre breads (min. 3 g fibre per slice)*
	Muffins/Doughnuts		
	Noodles (canned or instant)		
	Pancakes/Waffles		
	Pasta filled with cheese or meat		
	Pizza		
	Rice (short-grain, white, instant)		

* Limit serving size (see page 25).

LUNCH	RED	YELLOW		GREEN
Fruits/ Vege- tables (Fresh/ Frozen)	Broad beans	Apricots (fresh and dried)**	Apples	Olives*
	French fries	Artichokes	Arugula	Onions
	Melons	Bananas	Asparagus	Oranges (all varieties)
	Most dried fruit	Beets	Avocado*	Peaches
	Parsnips	Corn	Beans (green/wax)	Pears
	Potatoes (mashed or baked)	Kiwi	Bell peppers	Peas
	Rutabaga	Mango	Blackberries	Peppers (hot)
		Papaya	Blueberries	Pickles
		Pineapple	Broccoli	Plums
		Potatoes (boiled)	Brussels sprouts	Potatoes (boiled new or small)
		Squash	Cabbage	Radishes
		Sweet potatoes	Carrots	Raspberries
		Yams	Cauliflower	Snow peas
			Celery	Spinach
			Cherries	Strawberries
			Cucumbers	Tomatoes
			Eggplant	Zucchini
			Grapefruit	
			Grapes	
			Leeks	
			Lemons	
			Lettuce	

FATS			
	Butter	Mayonnaise (light)	Almonds*
	Hard margarine	Most nuts	Canola oil*
	Mayonnaise	Peanut butter (100% peanuts)	Mayonnaise (fat-free)
	Peanut butter (regular, light)	Peanut oil	Olive oil*

* Limit serving size (see page 25).
** For baking, it is acceptable to use a modest amount of dried apricots or cranberries.

LUNCH	RED	YELLOW	GREEN
	Salad dressings (regular)	Salad dressings (light)	Salad dressings (low-fat, low-sugar)
	Tropical oils	Soft margarine (non-hydrogenated)	Soft margarine (non-hydrogenated, light)*
SOUPS			
	All cream-based soups	Canned chicken noodle	Chunky bean and vegetable soups (e.g., Campbell's Healthy Request, Healthy Choice)
	Canned black bean	Canned lentil	Homemade soups with green-light ingredients
	Canned green pea	Canned tomato	
	Canned puréed vegetable		
	Canned split pea		

* Limit serving size (see page 25).

THE BROWN-BAG OPTION

Bringing your lunch to work is the easiest way to ensure you eat the green-light way. And there are other advantages to brown-bagging it: it's cheaper and it gives you extra downtime. If you prefer to eat out at a restaurant or fast-food outlet, turn to chapter 9.

SANDWICHES

No wonder sandwiches are the lunchtime staple: they are portable, easy to make and offer endless variety. Unfortunately, they can also be a dietary disaster, but if you follow the suggestions below, you can keep your sandwiches green-light.

● Always use whole wheat or whole-grain bread (minimum of 3 grams of fibre per slice).
● Sandwiches should be served open faced. To prevent the bread getting soggy, either pack components separately and assemble just before eating or make your sandwich with a "lettuce lining."

- Include at least three vegetables, such as lettuce, tomato, red or green bell peppers, cucumber, sprouts or onion. Instead of spreading the bread with butter or margarine, use mustard or hummus.
- Add up to 4 ounces of cooked lean meat or fish. If you make tuna or chicken salad, use low-fat mayonnaise or low-fat salad dressing and celery. Mix canned salmon with malt vinegar or fresh lemon.

SALADS

Invest in a variety of reusable glass containers so you can bring individual-sized salads to work. Keep a supply of green-light vinaigrette on hand and wash greens ahead of time and store in paper towels in plastic bags. You'll find that salads are a creative way to use up leftovers with a minimum of fuss.

You will find a series of salad suggestions in chapter 8.

SNACKS

Keep your digestive system busy and your energy up with three between-meal snacks daily.

Try three balanced snacks that include some protein and carbohydrates (e.g., a piece of fruit with a few nuts, or Laughing Cow light cheese with celery sticks).

You might also want to explore the world of food bars. Be careful when choosing as most are full of cereal and sugar. The ones to look for have a higher protein level. Half a Balance Bar or Zone Bar is an excellent snack. So are most bars that weigh between 50 and 65 grams and have around 200 calories and, most importantly, contain at least 12 grams of protein. Check labels carefully.

Keep in mind that many snacks and desserts labelled "low fat" or "sugar-free" are not necessarily green-light. Sugar-free instant pudding and "low-fat" muffins are still high G.I. because they contain highly processed grains.

If you bake your own green-light muffins and granola bars (the recipes are in chapter 8), they also make good snacks. You can freeze a batch or two and reheat them in the microwave.

SNACKS	RED	YELLOW	GREEN
	Bagels	Dark chocolate (70% cocoa)	Almonds*
	Candy	Ice cream (low-fat)	Applesauce (unsweetened)
	Cookies	Nuts (except those listed green-light)	Canned peaches/pears in juice or water
	Crackers	Popcorn (light, microwaveable)	Cottage cheese (1% or fat-free)
	Doughnuts		Extra-low-fat cheese (e.g., Laughing Cow Light, Boursin Light)
	Flavoured gelatin (all varieties)		Frozen yogurt (low-fat)
	French fries		Fruit yogurt 1/2 cup (fat-free with sweetener)
	Ice cream		Hazelnuts*
	Muffins (commercial)		Homemade green-light snacks (see pages 138–142)
	Popcorn (regular)		Ice cream 1/2 cup (low-fat and no added sugar)
	Potato chips		Most fresh/frozen fruit
	Pretzels		Most fresh/frozen vegetables
	Pudding		High protein bars**
	Raisins		Pickles
	Rice cakes		Pumpkin seeds
	Sorbet		Sugar-free hard candies
	Tortilla chips		Sunflower seeds
	Trail mix		
	White bread		

* Limit serving size (see page 25).
** 180-225 calorie bars, e.g. Zone or Balance Bars; 1/2 bar per serving.

DINNER

Dinner, traditionally, is the main meal of the day—and the one at which we may have a tendency to overeat. Unlike breakfast and lunch, dinner doesn't usually have any time or availability constraints (although juggling our schedules along with our children's can sometimes make this a moot point).

The typical North American dinner comprises three things: meat or fish, potato, pasta or rice, and vegetables. Together, these foods provide an assortment of carbohydrates, proteins and fats, along with other minerals and vitamins essential to our health.

(For a complete list of foods, see the Complete G.I. Diet Food Guide on page 183–92).

DINNER	RED	YELLOW	GREEN
PROTEIN			
Meat, Poultry, Fish, Eggs and Meat Substitutes	Breaded fish and seafood	Fish canned in oil	All fish and seafood, fresh, frozen (not breaded nor canned in oil)
	Ground beef (more than 10% fat)	Ground beef (lean)	Beef (lean cuts)
	Hamburgers	Lamb (lean cuts)	Chicken/Turkey breast (skinless)
	Hot dogs	Pork (lean cuts)	Egg whites
	Processed meats	Whole regular eggs (preferably omega-3)	Ground beef (extra-lean)
	Sausages	Chicken/turkey leg (skinless)	Lean deli ham
	Sushi		Liquid eggs (e.g., Break Free)
			Pork tenderloin
			Textured vegetable protein
			Tofu (soft)
			Veal

DINNER	RED	YELLOW	GREEN
Dairy	Almond milk	Cheese (light)	Buttermilk
	Cheese	Cream cheese (light)	Cottage cheese (1% or fat-free)
	Chocolate milk	Ice cream (low-fat)	Cream cheese (fat-free)
	Cottage cheese (whole or 2%)	Milk (1%)	Extra low-fat cheese (e.g., Laughing Cow Light, Boursin Light)
	Evaporated milk	Sour cream (light)	Frozen yogurt (1/2 cup, low-fat)
	Goat milk	Yogurt (low-fat)	Flavoured yogurt (non-fat with sweetener)
	Rice milk		Ice cream (1/2 cup, low-fat, no added sugar)
	Sour cream		Milk (skim)
	Yogurt (whole or 2%)		Sour cream (1% or less)
			Soy milk (plain, low-fat)
			Whey protein powder
CARBOHYDRATES			
Breads/ Grains	Bagels	Pita (whole wheat)	Pasta (fettuccine, spaghetti, penne, vermicelli, linguine, macaroni)*
	Baguette/Croissants	Whole-grain breads*	Quinoa
	Cake/Cookies		Rice (basmati, wild, brown, long-grain)*
	Macaroni and cheese		Whole-grain, high-fibre breads (min. 3g fibre per slice)*
	Muffins/Doughnuts		
	Noodles (canned or instant)		
	Pasta filled with cheese or meat		
	Pizza		
	Rice (short-grain, white, instant)		
	Tortillas		

DINNER	RED	YELLOW		GREEN	
Fruits/ Vegetables (Fresh/ Frozen)	Broad beans	Apricots		Apples	Lemons
	French fries	Bananas		Arugula	Lettuce
	Melons	Beets		Asparagus	Mushrooms
	Most dried fruit	Corn		Avocado*	Olives*
	Parsnips	Kiwi		Beans (green/wax)	Onions
	Potatoes (mashed or baked)	Mango		Bell peppers	Oranges (all varieties)
		Papaya		Blackberries	Peaches
		Pineapple		Blueberries	Pears
		Potatoes (boiled)		Broccoli	Peas
		Squash		Brussels sprouts	Peppers (hot)
		Sweet potatoes		Cabbage	Pickles
		Yams		Carrots	Plums
				Cauliflower	Potatoes (boiled, new or small)
				Celery	Radishes
				Cherries	Raspberries
				Cucumbers	Snow peas
				Eggplant	Spinach
				Grapefruit	Strawberries
				Grapes	Tomatoes
				Leeks	Zucchini

FATS				
	Butter	Mayonnaise (light)	Almonds*	
	Hard margarine	Most nuts	Canola oil*	
	Mayonnaise	Salad dressings (light)	Hazelnuts	
	Peanut butter (regular, light)	Soft margarine (non-hydrogenated)	Mayonnaise (fat-free)	
	Salad dressings (regular)	Vegetable oils	Olive oil*	
	Tropical oils	Walnuts	Pistachios*	

DINNER	RED	YELLOW	GREEN
	Vegetable shortening	Salad dressings (light)	Salad dressings (low-fat, low-sugar)
	Salad dressings (regular)	Soft margarine (non-hydrogenated)	Soft margarine (non-hydrogenated, light)*
	Tropical oils		Vegetable oil sprays
			Vinaigrette
Soups			
	All cream-based soups	Canned chicken noodle	Chunky bean and vegetable soups (e.g., Campbell's Healthy Request, Healthy Choice)
	Canned black bean	Canned lentil	Homemade soups with green-light ingredients
	Canned green pea	Canned tomato	
	Canned puréed vegetable		
	Canned split pea		
* Limit serving size (see page 25).			

PROTEIN

No dinner is complete without protein; whether it is in the form of meat, poultry, seafood, beans or tofu, it should cover no more than one-quarter of your plate and the serving size should be 4 ounces—roughly the size of the palm of your hand. Another good visual is a pack of cards, or so my friends with small palms tell me!

Red Meat

Most red meats contain saturated (bad) fat, so it's important to buy lean cuts or trim off all the visible fat. A loin steak trimmed to only a quarter-inch of fat can have up to half the fat of a steak with no trim.

Buy only low-fat meats such as top round beef, veal and pork tenderloin. Broiling or grilling allows the excess fat from the meat to drain off.

Poultry

Chicken and turkey breasts are excellent choices provided all the skin is removed. Skinless thighs, wings and legs are higher in fat and are therefore yellow-light.

Seafood

Fish and seafood are also excellent choices unless they've been breaded. Though certain fish, such as salmon, have a relatively high oil content, this omega-3 oil is extremely beneficial to your health, especially heart health.

● In terms of quantity, the best measure for meat or fish is your palm. As mentioned above, the portion should be about the size of the palm of your hand and about as thick.

Vegetarian

Beans and tofu are excellent sources of protein and you don't have to be a vegetarian to enjoy them. In fact, beans are nearly the perfect food; they not only contain protein but also are low in fat and high in fibre. Add them to salads and soups.

Although tofu is not a lot of fun in itself, it takes on the flavours of seasonings and cooking sauces. Choose soft tofu, which has up to one-third less fat than the firm variety. I am particularly impressed with another soy product, textured vegetable protein (TVP), which looks like, and can be used in the same way, as ground beef.

POTATOES

The G.I. rating of potatoes ranges from moderate to high, depending on the type and how they are cooked and served. In the lowest G.I. category are boiled, small (preferably new) potatoes served whole or sliced, two to three per serving. All other versions are strictly red-light.

PASTA

As mentioned earlier, the serving size is critical. Pasta should be a side dish and not form the base of the meal. Whole wheat pasta is preferable and is now widely available. Allow 3/4 cup cooked, per serving.

RICE

Rice has a broad G.I. range. The best choices are basmati, wild, brown or long-grain. These rices contain a starch, amylose, that breaks down more slowly than other rices. Again, serving size is critical. Allow three tablespoons of dry rice per serving, or 2/3 cup cooked.

Potatoes, pasta and rice should cover only one-quarter of your plate.

VEGETABLES/SALADS

This is where you can go wild. Eat as many vegetables and as much salad as you like. In fact, this should be the backbone of your meal. Virtually all vegetables are ideal. Remember that the best way to cook vegetables is to steam or microwave them until tender-crisp. Try to have a side salad with your daily dinner.

Watch out for salad dressings. Use only low-fat and fat-free ones, and check sugar content as manufacturers often bump up the sugar as they reduce the fat.

Serve two or three varieties of vegetables for dinner. Family-sized frozen bags of mixed, unseasoned vegetables are as nutritious as fresh and are convenient and relatively inexpensive.

DESSERTS

This is one of the most troublesome issues in any weight-control program. Desserts usually taste great, but they tend to be loaded with sugar and fat—a real guilt-inducing situation! As the last course in most meals, desserts often fall into the "Should I or shouldn't I?" category.

The good news is that dessert should be a part of your meal. There are a broad range of low-G.I., low-calorie alternatives that taste great and are good for you. Virtually any fruit qualifies (though hold off on the bananas and raisins) and there are numerous low-fat, low-sugar dairy products such as yogurt and ice cream. You won't be eating apple pie à la mode, but you could be enjoying applesauce with yogurt, or even a meringue with fresh or frozen berries.

WHAT CAN I DRINK?

Since 70 percent of our body is made up of water, it's hardly surprising that drinking fluids is an important part of any dietary program. Most dieticians recommend eight glasses of fluid per day. Don't feel you have to drink eight glasses of water a day *in addition* to other beverages. Milk, tea and soft drinks all contribute to the eight-glasses-a-day recommendation.

So the rule of thumb is to drink a glass of water with each of your three main meals and with each snack.

Because liquids don't trip satiety mechanisms, it's a waste taking in calories through them.

So what to drink?

WATER

The cheapest and best choice is plain, simple water. Try to drink an 8-ounce glass of water *before* each meal for two reasons. First, having your stomach partially filled with liquid before the meal means you will feel full more quickly, thus reducing the temptation to overeat. Second, you won't be tempted to "wash down" your food before it's been sufficiently chewed, thus upsetting your digestive system.

SOFT DRINKS

Sugar-free soft drinks are fine but make sure they are caffeine-free. Remember, caffeine effectively stimulates appetite.

SKIM MILK

This is my personal choice for breakfast and lunch. It's an excellent source of protein, which helps ensure you eat a balanced lunch in particular.

COFFEE

As I mentioned earlier, the principal problem with coffee is caffeine. Caffeine can stimulate insulin production, which encourages appetite. If you can't start your day without a cup, by all means go ahead and have one. But make sure it's just one cup per day.

Decaffeinated coffee is an ideal alternative especially with all the delicious new flavours now available in most supermarkets.

TEA

Tea has considerably less caffeine than coffee, and both black and green teas contain an antioxidant property that appears to carry significant heart health benefits. Tea has higher quantities of flavonoids (antioxidants) than any vegetable tested. Maybe my 100-year-old mother and her tea-drinking cronies are on to something!

FRUIT DRINKS/JUICES

Fruit drinks contain a large amount of sugar, are calorie-dense and are definitely red-light.

Fruit *juices* are preferable to fruit drinks, but as discussed earlier, it's always better to eat the fruit or vegetable rather than drink its juice. Juice contains less nutrition and more calories than the original fruit or vegetable and has a higher G.I.

ALCOHOL

This is a good news/bad news story. The good news is that alcohol in moderation—particularly red wine—is not only acceptable, but also can even be good for your health (see page 56).

The bad news is that alcohol is a disaster for weight control. Alcohol is easily metabolized by the body, which means increased insulin production leading to a drop in blood sugar levels. Your body then seeks more alcohol or food to boost those sagging sugar levels. This vicious circle can play havoc with your weight-loss plan. To make things worse, most alcoholic drinks are loaded with empty calories.

So no alcohol at all in Phase I.

THE FAMILY

One of the most frequent questions I am asked is whether the G.I. Diet is suitable for all members of the family, including children—and indeed it is. Phase II is a healthy way to eat for everyone, even if they don't need to lose any weight. Phase I is recommended for anyone who needs to reduce. If you think your child may be overweight, it is critical that you get your doctor's confirmation. Kids often put on weight prior to a growth spurt, and it's not something you should necessarily worry about. However, childhood obesity in this country has tripled over the past twenty-five years, so it's important to introduce children to good eating habits. Children should always eat a nutritious breakfast (not sugary cereals), lunch, dinner and snacks made up of green- and yellow-light foods. Fresh fruit, vegetables, chicken, fish, yogurt, whole wheat bread, pasta, porridge and nuts are all kid-friendly foods that will see to their nutritional needs. Remember that growing children need sufficient fat in their diet—the good kind found in nuts, fish and vegetable oils.

If your doctor agrees that your child is overweight, gently introduce him or her to the Phase I way of eating. Don't put pressure on children to lose weight, simply encourage healthy food choices. And allow them to enjoy special treats on holidays and occasions such as birthdays and Halloween.

VEGETARIANS

I was surprised at the number of vegetarians who wrote me asking whether the G.I. Diet was right for them. Most vegetarians I know don't need to lose weight. But if you do, the G.I. Diet is certainly the program for you. Just continue to substitute vegetable protein for animal protein—something you've been doing all along. However, because most vegetable protein sources, such as beans, are encased in fibre, your digestive system may not be getting the maximum protein benefit. So try to add easily digestible protein boosters like tofu and soy/whey protein powder.

You will find several vegetarian recipes in chapter 8, as well as suggestions on how to convert some recipes with meat to meatless.

Chapter Five
Ready, Set, Go!

READY

By now, I hope you understand the principles of the G.I. Diet and are totally convinced that the plan is going to work for you for the rest of your life. All that's left is to take the plunge. This is what I call the READY stage, and it is perhaps the most agonizing part of the journey.

The best advice I can give comes from my own experience. I knew I had to lose twenty pounds to take me to the 22 BMI target weight. On the advice of a friend I gathered together a number of books (diet books!) and piled them on my bathroom scale until they totalled twenty pounds. I then put them in a backpack and carried them around the house one Sunday morning. By noon the weight was really bugging me. What a relief it was to take the bag off my back! So the question was, did I want to carry that excess twenty pounds of fat around with me each and every day, or lose it and gain the sense of lightness and freedom I experienced after the backpack came off?

I urge you to try the same exercise. Identify how much weight you want to lose by using the BMI chart on pages 16–17. Rather than bundling up books, which can be rather bulky if you have a lot of weight to lose, fill some empty plastic bottles with water to equal that weight and carry them on your back or shoulder, or around your waist, for a few hours. Remember, that's the excess weight you are permanently carrying around with you. No wonder you feel exhausted! And that's one of the principal benefits of the G.I. Diet: not only will you look and feel great, but you will rediscover all that energy and zip you had in your teens and twenties, which you thought had been lost forever.

SET

Wondering what to do first? Well, let me suggest that you proceed in the following manner:

1. BASELINE

Before you do anything else, get your vital statistics on record. Measuring progress is a great motivator. Keep a log of your weekly progress in your bathroom where it's handy (see removable log sheet on page 198). There are two key measurements. The first is weight. Always weigh yourself at the same time of day, because a meal or bowel movement can throw out your weight by a couple of pounds. First thing in the morning, before you eat breakfast, is a good time. The other important measurement is your waist. Measure at your natural waistline—usually just above the navel while standing in a relaxed, normal posture. The tape should be snug but not indenting the skin.

Record both measurements on the bathroom log. I've added a Comments column to the log sheet where you can note how you're feeling, or any unusual events in the past week that might have some bearing on your progress.

2. PANTRY

Clear out your pantry, fridge and freezer of all red- and yellow-light products. Give them to a food bank or to your skinny neighbours. If the products aren't around, you won't be tempted to eat or drink them.

3. SHOPPING

Stock up at home on green-light products. You will find a shopping list on pages 193–95 to refer to at the grocery store. There are a few yellow-light products that have been asterisked, and these can be used sparingly during your Phase I weight-loss period. After a couple of shopping trips, selecting the right products will become second nature.

An important tip: make sure you don't go shopping on an empty stomach or you may make some poor food choices.

Although we've tried to provide a broad range of products, we could not hope to cover all the thousands of brands available in most supermarkets. As a result, we list foods by their generic name, e.g., "oatmeal," not "Quaker oatmeal." In today's competitive marketplace, most brands in any given category have similar formulations so your choice will usually be made on quality and taste. In the rare instances where there may be some variations in content between brands—bread is a good example—you may want to check out the nutritional labels. Look for six key numbers:

Nutrition Facts
Valeur nutritive

Serving 1 cup (55 g)
Portion de 1 tasse (55 g)

Amount Per Serving Teneur par portion	% Daily Value % valeur quotidienne
Calories / Calories 190	
Fat / Lipides 1.5 g	**2** %
Saturated / saturés 0 g + Trans / trans 0 g	**0** %
Cholesterol / Cholestérol 0 mg	**0** %
Sodium / Sodium 90 mg	**4** %
Potassium / Potassium 500 mg	**14** %
Carbohydrate / Glucides 31 g	**10** %
Fibre / Fibres 10 g	**42** %
Sugars / Sucres 6 g	
Protein / Protéines 14 g	
Vitamin A / Vitamine A	0 %
Vitamin C / Vitamine C	0 %
Calcium / Calcium	6 %
Iron / Fer	15 %
Phosphorus / Phosphore	20 %

1. **Serving size:** Is this realistic? Often manufacturers who are concerned about the fat, cholesterol or calories of that product will identify a serving size smaller than is realistic. You'll see this on the labels of many high-sugar cereals.

2. **Calories:** Remember that this number is based on the serving size; the lower the better.

3. **Fat:** Look for the product with the lower fat serving, particularly in terms of saturated and trans fat.

4. **Fibre:** Since fibrous foods have a lower G.I., look for the higher number of fibre grams per serving.

5. **Sugar:** Choose brands that are lower in sugar. Watch for products advertised as low fat where the manufacturer has bumped up the sugar content to make up for any perceived loss of taste. Yogurts and cereals are good examples.

    Sugars are sometimes listed as dextrose, glucose, fructose or sucrose; regardless of the form, they contain the same number of calories as sugar. Similarly, sugar alcohols—those ending in "–tol," such as sorbitol or maltitol—contain around 60 to 70 percent sugar. However, as they are correspondingly less sweet, manufacturers tend to boost their levels, meaning there is no net calorie gain over sugar. Avoid these.

6. **Sodium (salt):** Sodium increases water retention, which doesn't help when you're trying to lose weight. It also contributes to premenstrual bloating and is a factor in hypertension (high blood pressure). Combining high blood pressure with excess weight substantially raises your risk of heart disease and stroke. We currently consume more than twice the amount of salt recommended for a healthy diet.

When choosing between brands, read the labels and choose those which offer lower calories, fat (especially saturated), sugar, and sodium and those that are higher in fibre. That's the formula for all green-light products. By eating these foods you will reduce your calorie intake without going hungry.

You will be buying considerably more fruit and vegetables than previously, so be a little daring and try some varieties that are new to you. There's a wonderful world of fresh and frozen produce just waiting for you to enjoy!

Remember: don't go food shopping with an empty stomach or you'll end up buying items that don't belong on the G.I. Diet!

GO

Now that the difficult part is done, it's plain sailing from here. Don't be surprised if you lose more than one pound per week in the first few weeks, as your body adjusts to the new regimen. Most of that weight will be water, not fat. Remember, 70 percent of our body weight is water.

Don't worry if from time to time you "fall off the wagon," eating or drinking with friends and going outside the program. That's the real world, and though it will marginally delay your target date, it's more important that you not feel as though you're living in a straitjacket. You should aim to live about 90 percent within the program and 10 percent outside. You will feel better and more energized when on the program and rarely feel deprived. However, in Phase I, try to keep these lapses to a minimum; you will be able to allow yourself more leeway once you have achieved your target weight.

If you want further proof or reassurance that your new way of eating is really working, try this test. After a couple of months on the G.I. Diet, break all the rules and have a lunch consisting of a whole pizza with the works, a bread roll and a beer or regular soft drink. While you're at it, finish up with a slice of pie. I'll spare you the ice cream.

I did just that, and by about three in the afternoon I could hardly keep awake. I felt listless and worn out. I hadn't planned on eating so much but got caught up in a fellow employee's farewell lunch. The reason for my afternoon fatigue (which you've likely figured out for yourself) was the combination of high-G.I. foods (pizza, bread roll, beer and pie), which led to a rapid spike in my blood sugar level. The resulting rush of insulin drained this sugar from my blood and caused my sugar levels to drop precipitously, leaving my brain and muscles starved of energy, i.e., in a hypoglycemic state. No wonder I couldn't keep my eyes open. I resolved then and there never to let this happen again! Though we will be talking about motivation in chapter 11, here are some tips to keep you motivated, especially when your resolve starts flagging (as it inevitably will from time to time):

1. Maintain a weekly progress log. Nothing is more motivating than success.
2. Set up a reward system. Buy yourself a small gift when you achieve a predetermined weight goal—perhaps a gift for every three pounds lost.
3. Identify family members or friends who will be your cheerleaders. Make them active participants in your plan. Even better, find a friend who will join the plan for mutual support.
4. Avoid acquaintances and haunts that may encourage your old behaviours. You know who I mean!
5. For women, try adding what a friend calls a special "spa" day to your week—a day when you are especially good with your program. This gives you some extra credit in your weight-loss account to draw on when the inevitable relapse occurs.
6. Keep up-to-date on the latest developments in diet and health at our website, www.gidiet.com.

Chapter Six
Phase II

Congratulations! You've achieved your new weight target!

This may be hard to believe, but when I had reached my target weight—I had lost 22 pounds, and 4 inches off my waist—I had to make a conscious effort to eat more in order to avoid losing more weight. My wife said I was entering the "gaunt zone"!

PHASE II MEALS AND SNACKS

The objective in Phase II is to increase the number of calories you consume so that you maintain your new weight. Remember the equation: food energy ingested must equal energy expended to keep weight stable. During Phase I you were taking in less food energy than you were expending, using your fat reserves to make up the shortfall. Now we make up that deficit by taking in some extra food energy, or calories.

Two words of caution. First, your body has become accustomed to doing with fewer calories and has, to a certain extent, adapted. The result is that your body is more efficient than in the bad old days when it had more food energy than it could use. Second, your new lower weight requires fewer calories to function. For example, if you lost 10 percent of your weight, then you need 10 percent fewer calories for your body to function.

Combining a more efficient body, which requires less energy to operate, with a lower weight, which requires fewer calories, means that you need only a marginal increase in food energy to balance the energy in/energy out equation. The biggest mistake most people make when coming off a diet is assuming that they can now consume a much higher calorie level than their new body really needs. The bottom line is that Phase II is only marginally different from Phase I. Phase II provides you with an opportunity to make small adjustments to portion size and add new foods from the yellow-light category. All the fundamentals of the Phase I plan, however, remain inviolable. The following are some suggestions for how you might wish to modify your new eating pattern in Phase II:

BREAKFAST
- Increase cereal serving size, e.g., from 1/2 to 2/3 cup oatmeal.
- Add a slice of 100% whole-grain toast and a pat of margarine.
- Double up on the sliced almonds on cereals.
- Help yourself to an extra slice of back bacon.
- Have a glass of juice now and then.
- Add a yellow-light fruit—a banana or apricots—to your cereal.
- Have a fully caffeinated coffee. Try to limit yourself to one a day, and make sure it's a good one!

LUNCH
I suggest you continue to eat lunch as you did in Phase I. This is the one meal that contained some compromises in the weight-loss portion of the program, since it is a meal most of us buy each day.

DINNER
- Add another boiled, preferably new, potato (from 2 or 3 to 3 or 4).
- Increase the rice or pasta serving from 6 to 1 cup.
- Have a 6-ounce steak instead of your regular 4 ounce. Make this a special treat, not a habit.
- Eat a few more olives and nuts, but watch the serving size as these are calorie heavyweights.
- Try a cob of sweet corn with a dab of non-hydrogenated margarine.

- Add a slice of whole-grain, high-fibre bread.
- Try a lean cut of lamb or pork (maximum 4-ounce serving).
- Have a glass of red wine with dinner.

SNACKS
Warning: Strictly watch quantity or serving size.
- Light microwave popcorn (maximum 2 cups).
- Nuts, maximum 10 to 12.
- A square or two of bittersweet chocolate (see below).
- A banana.
- One tablespoon of 100% peanut butter.

CHOCOLATE
To many of us, the idea of a chocolate-free world is abhorrent. The good news is that some chocolate, in limited quantities, is acceptable.

Most chocolate contains large quantities of saturated fat and sugar, making it quite fattening. However, chocolate with a high cocoa content (70 percent) delivers more chocolate satisfaction per ounce. So, a square or two of rich, dark, bittersweet chocolate, nibbled slowly or, better yet, dissolved in the mouth, gives us chocoholics just the fix we need. This high-cocoa chocolate is available at most drug stores and supermarkets.

ALCOHOL
Now is the moment some of you have been waiting for. In Phase II a daily glass of wine, preferably red and with dinner, is not only allowed—it's encouraged! Recently, there has been a flood of research into the benefits of alcohol on personal health. It is generally agreed that some alcohol is better than none at all, especially for heart health. It has been found that red wine in particular is rich in flavonoids and, when drunk in moderation (a glass a day), has a demonstrable benefit in reducing the risk of heart attack and

stroke. The theory that says if one glass is good for you, two must be better is tempting but not true. One glass gives the optimum benefit.

As with coffee, if you're only going to have a glass of wine a day, make it a great one.

My eldest son, who is a computer whiz in Seattle and lives a lifestyle I can only dream about, took me at my word about wine and gave me a subscription to the *Wine Spectator*. It has proven to be the most costly present I've ever received, as a whole new world of wine and wine ratings has opened up to me. My $10-a-bottle ceiling for special occasions has now doubled or tripled, though it has all been rationalized: I'm drinking less, so I can afford the extravagance!

As a beer aficionado, I like to drink the occasional beer as an alternative to wine. This habit has recently received an endorsement from a group of scientists who reported that beer (in moderation) would reduce cholesterol and thus heart disease, delay menopause, and reduce the risk of several cancers. They also noted that beer has anti-inflammatory and anti-allergic properties, plus a positive effect on bone density. Personally, I worry about any product being touted as the wonder cure for all our ills, but clearly a glass of beer with supper is likely to do little harm. Remember, though, that because of its high malt content, beer is a high-G.I. beverage, so moderation is particularly important.

If you do drink alcohol, always have it with your meal. Food slows down the absorption of alcohol, thereby minimizing its impact.

THE WAY YOU WILL EAT FOR THE REST OF YOUR LIFE

With all these new options in Phase II, the temptation may be to overdo it. If the pounds start to reappear, simply revert to the Phase I plan for a while and you'll be astonished at how quickly your equilibrium is restored.

Phase II is the way you will eat for the rest of your life. You will look and feel better, have more energy and experience none of those hypoglycemic lows. One reason, of course, that you have more energy is that you're not carrying around all that surplus fat. It might be fun to resurrect the backpack and load it up with the weight you've just lost. Carry it around on your back for an hour or two and then rejoice that you don't have to carry it around for the rest of your life! Whenever your resolve wavers, reach for the backpack. It's a marvellous motivator.

The opportunity to succeed is in your hands. I've tried to give you a simple yet motivating plan that will not leave you hungry, tired or confused. It's all here in the book; the rest is up to you.

So, put on the backpack for a couple of hours, clear out the pantry and drive to the supermarket. Remember to park as far as possible from the entrance and enjoy the extra walk. Everything starts with a first step!

Chapter Seven
Changing Behaviours

BY DR. RUTH GALLOP

INTRODUCTION

In this chapter Rick has asked me to write about how behaviour affects our eating behaviours. I will talk about three critical areas: how to identify and manage personality characteristics or traits that influence eating behaviours, eating behaviours for which we are all at risk, and emotional eating. In previous books I have written about emotional eating and the use of food as comfort. Now, in response to thousands of e-mails that have described both the successes and challenges of staying with the G.I. Diet due to behaviours associated with personality traits, I will look more closely at this issue and consider ways that people can use self-knowledge to modify their eating behaviours.

During my career I have spent much of my time teaching about how we develop our personalities and sense of self, and about how we bring psychological baggage from our childhoods with us into adulthood. Much as we would wish we could leave it parked outside at the curb, it just doesn't happen. Both nature (our genetic inheritance) and nurture (our upbringing) work together to make us who we are. While each one of us is unique, certain basic personality characteristics can be widely observed in the population. Unfortunately, trying to change these characteristics is extremely difficult. For years I have tried to help health care professionals recognize that just because they and/or their clients would like to change behaviour doesn't mean it will necessarily happen. So teaching about *how* to help individuals change behaviours has been at the core of my work.

HOW WE RESPOND

Thousands of people want to lose weight. They may feel bad or guilty, and are often anxious and suffer from low self-esteem. They want to be successful; however, they bring to weight-loss efforts their own personality traits and associated eating behaviours. And it is these eating behaviours that need to be addressed if success is to be achieved.

If we could change behaviours easily then weight control would be simple. But behaviours are simply the expression of traits that determine how we will respond to situations. When we are placed in any situation that arouses conflict, we have a response. As you will see, it can take differing forms. For example, when offered a chocolate, your first thought might be, "Oh, my favourite, chocolate!" (The next thought might be, "If I eat it, it will go straight to my hips" followed by, "Well, why should I deprive myself?" Next, feelings start to interfere: "I hate this—why can't have what I want? It's so unfair, *other* people don't agonize over a simple piece of chocolate." You start feeling bad; maybe even your pulse increases or you feel anxious. And in the end you end up eating too many chocolates, then immediately beat yourself up—until the next time it happens.)

That's just one type of reaction. Another person might be offered the same chocolate and think, "She knows I'm trying to lose weight—why is she doing this to me?" Another might think, "One won't do any harm," and so on. Each situation will generate its own response set of thoughts, associated feelings, physical arousal and behaviours. Behaviours are the end point of each sequence and may generate the next round.

These response sequences are not chance events; you respond with a variation of your own types of responses every time you are confronted with a conflict situation. This sequence is your own characteristic trait, and changing that sequence requires awareness and effort.

For better or worse, weight, particularly for women, has

a lot to do with self-esteem. Our society sends the message that feeling attractive is essential. We are bombarded daily with ways to look younger, slimmer and sexier. As we mature, our bodies change: at first we get curves; then we may or may not have children, and then we hit menopause and the curves rearrange themselves in ways we might not choose. And through life's journey, many women struggle to keep their weight under control. It is that sense of control that we strive to attain in other areas of our lives because we so often associate it with feeling successful and satisfied.

For men, weight control is usually about health; men are less conscious of appearance. In fact, some men strut proudly on the beach leading with their beer bellies! But often as men age and weight creeps up, health risks start to build—type two diabetes, heart and joint problems are all associated with weight and age. But men don't want to think about this—for men, self-esteem is associated with virility and being in charge. Having to worry about weight is thought of as a more female preoccupation, and implies a loss of control and a loss of masculinity. So denial, excuse making and rationalizing are often traits that men display when dealing with their eating issues.

Our personality style is our glue—it holds us together; it influences how we deal with people and how we deal with challenges at home and at work. Our personality also reflects the way we maintain our sense of control—and the issue of control plays a dominant role in how we deal with food and the challenges of weight loss and maintenance. The goal of the personality section of this book is to help you learn about the particular style that directs your personal eating behaviours and be able to modify those behaviours and take control.

I have a friend I'll call Sue, who fears she will eat the whole box of maple fudge if put in front of her—and her fear is quite real. In fact, the fear of being out of control structures

Sue's life: she always knows what she'll be doing and when she'll be doing it, her cupboards are super neat and her success as a senior administrator actually depends on her organizational abilities. And, as for the fudge, she manages by never going near it. In this way, as with other areas in her life, she minimizes the potential anxiety she associates with loss of control. But she had to recognize this about herself, which was an absolutely essential first step. Once Sue had self-awareness, she was able to be in charge of her life. Sue knows that order and control soothes and relieves her anxiety so she can purposefully determine how much or how little control she needs in each situation.

On the other hand, another mutual friend wishes she could be more like Sue in the organization department, and occasionally tries to discipline herself by making lists and menu plans. Some of her efforts have borne fruit: for example, when cooking, she used to always be dashing around her kitchen, finding she was out of an ingredient, or forgetting a crucial component or step. So she made a conscious effort always to put out all her ingredients and tools before starting, and thus managed to change an ingrained behaviour. But in other endeavours, her resolve to change has ebbed after a short time, because it is hard to alter your basic traits.

Recognizing our own characteristics is not always straightforward. We often have overlapping characteristics although usually one personality pattern is likely to dominate.

We have grouped the behavioural characteristics of dieters into four categories.

- The Controller
- The Impulsive Eater
- The Procrastinator/Avoider
- The Eater with Self-Esteem Issues

To illustrate each of these personality characteristics, here are some excerpts from readers' letters as they struggle to take control over their eating habits.

CONTROLLER

Vikrim: "I've followed your diet precisely, no cheating, kept a journal but I have not lost any weight in the last three days—what is wrong?"

IMPULSIVE

Debra: "We were on vacation we had sausages and eggs for breakfast . . . and a bag of mint Oreo cookies and ice cream in drinks . . . Part of me says I'm over sixty and what the hell, I want to enjoy life, yet another part of me knows that if I don't get it under control I won't have much life left to enjoy . . ."

PROCRASTINATOR/AVOIDER

June: "I like to stay on target but when I come home at the end of the day or week of work I have no energy to go shopping or prepare a healthy meal—so I put it off until next week."

With this person, the excuse is sometimes covered by an apparent qualified endorsement: a "yes but" approach, which is reflected in what Ann says:

"I'm sure this is an excellent way to lose weight but I have trouble with some foods with fibre or soy so I don't think this one is for me."

SELF-ESTEEM ISSUES

Metha: "As a child, my sister was 'the beautiful one' and I was 'the smart one.' My parents adored her and treated me differently. Food filled a void and I hid behind people in every photo so that I was just a head—never a body."

WHO ARE YOU?

Find out which personality characteristics or traits best describe you. How much value this book will be for you will largely depend on how honest you are in your answers. I want to stress **there are no right or wrong choices.** These traits are neither good nor bad—they are just part of who we are. The more we know and understand ourselves, the more empowered we feel.

Check the items that describe you.

THE CONTROLLER C

Worried about losing control, Controllers monitor everything, which can drive themselves and everyone around them crazy. Foods are weighed, counted and watched. Controllers often have an encyclopedic knowledge of calories, carbs, etc., and often eating is devoid of any pleasure.

- I watch what I eat very carefully.
- I keep careful records or food diaries
- I like to know the caloric/carbohydrate content of all food.
- I create detailed weekly menus.
- I am very organized.
- I am very neat.
- I don't like clutter or disorganized spaces.
- I rarely do activities spontaneously.
  TOTAL _____

THE IMPULSIVE EATER IE

Impulsive eaters act before they think. Life is often devoid of order and driven by moment to moment decisions. Often there is much regret about past actions.

- I eat secretly.
- I sometimes lie about what I have eaten.
- I overindulge at buffets.

- I can never stop at just one chocolate, cookie, etc.
- I keep cookies on hand, or ice cream in freezer—just in case.
- When I go out for a coffee I'll have a muffin or pastry even though I had planned to have just coffee.
- I keep candies or chocolate in my desk at work and eat some every day.
- In general I am an impulsive shopper.
- I often buy foods I wish I hadn't.
  TOTAL _____

Believe it or not, Controllers and Impulsive Eaters have similar traits. Both are struggling with issues of control: one fears losing control and the other fears being controlled—two sides of the same coin.

THE PROCRASTINATOR/AVOIDER PA

Mary has tried every diet under the sun. Each time she fails but explains that the failure rests not in her own behaviour but in something external. See if you identify with any of the statements in the following list.

- Following a diet is too complicated.
- My weight isn't a big problem anyway.
- My kids don't like the food and I can't be making different foods from the rest of the family.
- I don't have the time to cook.
- I travel for work and this doesn't work.
- I can't do this during the holidays, at Christmas, on vacation, at the relatives', etc.
- I ask for help or advice but it never quite fits my situation.
- I've tried everything anyone suggests and it hasn't worked for me.
- People get frustrated with me for no apparent reason.
  TOTAL _____

THE EATER WITH SELF-ESTEEM ISSUES (ESI)

This is a complicated one because it so often overlaps with emotional eating which will be discussed later in this chapter. These people eat poorly because they don't like themselves or don't think they are good enough.

- I'm not very attractive.
- People don't really like me.
- My sibling is smarter/more attractive than I am.
- I'm uncomfortable in social situations.
- I always disappoint people.
- I could never really please my parents.
- I'm not doing a good job parenting.
- I worry my partner will lose interest in me.
- Food is the main thing that makes me feel better.
  TOTAL _____

Having checked off which of the descriptors above best suit you, tally up the check marks. If you have checked off half or more in a category, it most likely best describes your personality type. You may well find that you fall into more than one category, but not to worry—many of us do not fit nicely into behavioural boxes. The important thing is to recognize and be aware of your own personal characteristics. Be honest. Procrastinator/avoiders can have trouble identifying themselves so if you kept thinking, "This is not really me," you know where you belong!

EATING BEHAVIOURS

We'll now take a closer look at these various characteristics and their associated behaviours and see how they relate to you taking charge of your diet and lifestyle.

THE CONTROLLER C

There's no denying that a certain degree of control is useful for maintaining weight and health. Having routines provides comfort, order and predictability in our lives. Knowing essentially how our day—and life—is structured is soothing. But, as is so often the way, too much of a good thing can be self-defeating. What happens when control issues take over every aspect of food and eating so that the very act of taking in nourishment becomes both stressful and a chore? When Rick designed the G.I. Diet, he was responding to the need to simplify weight-loss programs and avoid the weighing, counting and measuring that lead many people to give up before reaching their goal. The G.I. Diet has only a few serving-size restrictions, coupled with eating green-light foods in moderation. But this type of diet with its minimal rules can be anxiety provoking for Controllers.

While it is good to select healthy foods and make wise food decisions, we should not become so immobilized by food choices that we cannot choose what to eat without strict policing. But it's this very policing that prevents Controllers from eating moderately and being in real control. So Controllers need help in making eating more relaxed and pleasurable, easing up on the self-monitoring and still feeling sufficiently in control.

We hear from many readers who have kept strictly to the rules and find that after a few weeks they are not losing weight at the rate they expected or, even worse, they haven't lost weight in the past week and want to know what they are "doing wrong." This is typical thinking for Controllers, who want everything in a perfectly straight line: you go on a diet, you follow the rules and the weight comes off. But since life and the human condition are not nice and orderly, deviations will occur. For Controllers, this is a game stopper. After a while the rigidity required to police oneself continuously gets boring and exhausting. When Controllers give up it's because they feel hungry, tired and deprived. The result is that they lose control by binging or overeating and the cycle starts again.

Here is an e-mail from a reader. "Every day for each of my snacks, I have an eight-ounce glass of water, nuts, an egg white, a piece of fruit and a radish. Would that be the right amount of protein per snack? As for the nuts, I always have eight per snack. Is that too many? (The radish and the egg white are both cut in half; one half of a radish goes inside one egg white half. I secure that with a toothpick, and there I have two hors-d'oeuvres for my snack.)." So this very precise eater wants even more rules! How long can the reader maintain this before becoming bored with her snack and tired of being so careful?

So people in this category need to be able to relax a little and function with less rigidity and fewer rules. The first step requires honest recognition that this is you. Make a long list of green-light foods you can eat, with very few limits on specific amounts and then make your meals from that list. We want you to have three meals and three snacks, and we want you to select foods you really like from the list for these meals, eating slowly and enjoying the foods. No careful measuring, counting, no food journal. Shift your focus from the control and the additional rules you create for yourself and try to experience the sensations attached to eating. Make up a week's list of meals you will like—we'll provide some sample weeks at the end of this book—but you must make some changes to specific likes of your own. This will provide sufficient structure and lots of variety. Enjoy the week—and each day consider whether you really savoured your meals. If you didn't, what Controller behaviour was interfering? How can you lighten up and still stay with the program? Congratulate yourself for being able to eat without measuring and chaos or binging did not result.

If planning for a whole week is too uncomfortable, take one day of meals and snacks—no measuring, no counting, and no weighing of food. Just be reasonable and go for green-light foods. For example:

- A small handful of nuts.
- A bunch of greens.
- A small piece of chicken or fish.
- A few boiled, small new potatoes.

Notice I'm using descriptive words for size, not specific quantities. Is it tolerable? Too much anxiety? Try one meal per day to start.

Try going to a buffet. Look for green-light foods you like, and have some (there's that unquantifiable word again). Fill your plate—eat and enjoy. If you are at a celebration and see your favourite red-light dessert—have a piece and enjoy. In fact, I would like you to have a small serving of a favourite forbidden food two or three times a week. Just do it—give yourself permission and don't think twice about it. What is the worst thing that can happen? If one day you eat too much, it's not a catastrophe—the next day you'll be back on the wagon. Occasional lapses happen to all of us—just get going again. If you have particular weaknesses that frighten you—such as chocolates or potato chips, then keep them out of the house or do what we will suggest for impulsive eaters, and make up small bags of these dangerous treats. Eat one bag as a snack; slowly savouring your favourite taste.

In summary:

- Recognize that control is an expression of fear of the loss of control.
- Ease up on rules.
- Try to enjoy eating.
- Minimize measuring and counting.
- Use descriptive measures such as "small," "moderate," "a handful."
- Focus on eating the green-light foods you like.
- Have occasional red-light treats and discover that disaster does not follow.
- Keep foods you fear out of the home and workplace.

THE IMPULSIVE EATER (IE)

In contrast to Controllers, Impulsive Eaters (IEs) don't want to think about food rules and don't want to be controlled by a perceived external controller. IEs fear control. Perhaps when growing up they experienced many food rules at home or their choices were always criticized. Better to make no choices now—as a result, IEs act impulsively. Often IEs mask this behaviour by declaring they are free spirits who answer to no one; however, they are just fleeing from fears of making bad choices.

So how do you start to think about impulsive eating? First you need to recognize that your impulsive eating is about a fear of being criticized for choices and being controlled. Ironically, the way to deal with it is by taking control yourself. This means consciously acknowledging, "I eat because I don't like people telling me what to do or criticizing what I do—either in my home, work, personal life, etc. I may have to follow rules in some areas of my life, but in my eating I can be in control and make my own choices. I can deliberately and purposefully choose to eat reasonably. No one will take my food away. I can choose what I want to eat today and what I want to eat tomorrow. The choices are mine, and I am in charge."

That last sentence must be your mantra—and it may need to be repeated daily.

Practically, IEs need to realize that grazing is a highly risky behaviour usually involving unconscious eating. Every passing of the fridge is an opportunity to check inside for a little something. The same goes for that "treat drawer" in your desk at work or at home. Make some notes on how often you graze during a day and analyze whether you were hungry at the time. Before you choose to have a snack, ask yourself, "Do I really need to eat that right now? Can I wait twenty minutes and see what happens?" (Likely you'll be busy with something else and will be that much closer to mealtime or your next real snack time). Sometimes something as simple as a glass of water (plain or carbonated) is sufficient to delay the urge.

Avoid eating out of bags (e.g., bags of nuts, chips, etc.). Make up individual snack-size bags and put the rest out of sight. Do this for all your snack food—muffins, nuts, popcorn, veggies, etc.—if you think it will help.

Plan your meals and brown-bag green-light food for lunch. Carry high-protein bars in your purse so a half bar is always available for an emergency snack when caught away from home. It will save you from a high-calorie muffin or Danish!

When you are preparing foods, follow serving-size guidelines.

Avoid eating in front of the TV—IEs can chow down vast amounts of food without being aware of amounts. If you really enjoy eating and watching TV and don't think you can manage without it, then use one of your premeasured snacks. Otherwise, try to find a different activity, such as scrapbooking or knitting, that you like to do with your hands while watching TV.

Keep all red-light food out of the house and out of your work desk or work site.

Do not use treats as a reward—this is self-defeating and will lead to more impulsive eating and ultimately giving up.

When at buffets, plan your approach. Scan the foods and make the decision to go up only once. First fill half your plate with salad and then fill the other half with green-light foods you enjoy. Have dessert if you want it—decide which your favourite is and have a small piece. Do **not** deny yourself dessert—you will feel resentful and this can set you onto the path of, "I deserve dessert—I'm going to have whatever I want . . ."

In summary:

- Recognize impulsive eating is fear of being controlled.
- Choices are yours to make.
- Avoid grazing.
- Have measured snacks—never eat out of a bag or jar.
- Avoid eating in front of the TV.
- Keep all red-light food out of house.

- Do not use food as a reward.
- Plan your approach to buffets.

THE PROCRASTINATOR/AVOIDER PA

Another way to avoid failure is to deny the problem, which is a common approach among men. Since many people trying to lose weight have tried different diets without success, failure is often something people know well. Like Impulsive Eaters, Procrastinators/Avoiders (PAs) are afraid of failure. They believe that it is better to never start at all than to start and fail. So rather than confront this fear of failure, they find reasons not to try and set up major hurdles to success.

PAs often use blame as a means of shifting the focus to an external source and away from themselves. Look back at the list of PA personality traits—many of the items on the list pinpoint the cause of the diet failure as something external, rather than actual eating behaviours. By not taking responsibility for the lack of action, PAs do not have to deal with personal failure. Someone or something has let them down. Usually this thinking is followed by the "if only" sequence: "If only I had enough time [or a supportive family ... or fewer dietary restrictions] I'd be successful." Taking ownership of these delaying tactics is hard, but it is essential.

Like IEs, PAs have to risk acknowledging the fear of failure while at the same time putting the risk of failure in proportion. Another major challenge for PAs (and to some extent IEs) is the wish for immediate impressive results. This is why so many fail on fad diets: in the beginning they seem to provide instant gratification—think of the thousands of magazine headlines that shout "Lose 15 pounds or three inches from your waist in ten days!" But when the diet proves unsustainable over the long term, what follows is a renewed sense of failure.

First, PAs need to set reasonable goals. If you have 50 pounds to lose then it is probably not realistic to start in May and assume you'll have lost all the weight in time for swimsuit season! Setting a goal of a pound a week is realistic—but to PAs, who crave instant results, it feels insignificant. So you have to recognize that it's a great week when you lose that pound, and that if you lose less or none at all the next week, it is *not* failure. It all averages out and patience is necessary. Not giving up when things don't go perfectly is tough but necessary.

Never have an extra treat with the plan and plan to make it up tomorrow by cutting back—it never works. Instead, eat properly one day at a time. And do make sure you're eating foods you really like. Eating should be a pleasure; you should not feel hard done by or suffer on the G.I. Diet. If you're not enjoying your food then you will use that as an excuse to quit.

Like IEs, PAs often eat when they are not hungry, and grazing during the day poses a real danger for PAs who are always ready to have a little extra something: "A small piece of cake can't do any harm and I'll skip dessert later." Work on grazing behaviour in small steps. Try to control grazing for one day at a time. Half-day goals won't work because you run the risk of blowing it in the afternoon and eating that piece of cake, which will provide an excuse to say, "I can't do it, I had to have that piece of cake—there is no point in trying." **Do not keep red-light treats of any kind in the workplace or home**. If you have a lapse, you need to acknowledge that one lapse doesn't justify giving up. PAs need to view each small success as a building block for the greater goal rather than view each small deviation as a failure and a reason to give up.

In summary:

- Recognize your fear of failure.
- Failure to start the diet or stick to it rests within the individual, not in external causes.
- The process of weight loss is slow and steady, not fast and furious.
- Recognize small successes that will accumulate into big successes.

- Never indulge today with the plan to restrict tomorrow.
- Eat green-light foods you enjoy in moderation.
- Eat when hungry—do not graze or watch TV when eating.
- Do not keep red-light foods in the workplace or home.
- One lapse does not justify quitting.

THE EATER WITH SELF-ESTEEM ISSUES ESI

Not feeling good about yourself in a fundamental way can permeate so many areas of your life. However, as we have heard from countless readers, when their bodies became slimmer and hence more attractive, they felt as if they were emerging from cocoons and rediscovering themselves. They not only had more energy and felt healthier but also felt able to participate in all sorts of activities and socializing. But how do you deal with years of feeling insecure or, as I tend to think of it feeling "not good enough"? Inside our heads we have all sorts of little judges ready to criticize us and prevent us from going forward. Even when friends and family tell us we are bright, attractive, intelligent, and so on, we feel they are only being nice.

I don't pretend that reading a couple of paragraphs will change your lifelong sense of self, but it's important to keep reinforcing some key facts. The evidence we have from people who have been successful suggests that self-worth can be significantly improved if you feel good about how you look. To care about how you look is not superficial or trivial—and it's not about some sort of Hollywood ideal, but just feeling comfortable and happy with your body image.

Eaters with Self-esteem Issues (ESIs) have often spent years serving others. Constantly putting aside one's own desires sometimes leads to a breakthrough of frustration or rage. ESIs are fearful that if they assert themselves others will abandon them. This false belief that they can hold the attention or friendship of others only by compromise and putting aside their wishes is so fundamental that asserting an opposing opinion or saying no to something carries with it both the risk of hurting feelings and the terrifying fear of abandonment. The ESIs are so sensitive to the experience of being hurt that the last thing they want to do is hurt someone's feelings. The reality is that the sensitivity lies with ESIs, not the receiver of their refusal.

Going on the G.I. Diet means putting your own self-interest first and that can be quite scary. The reality is that if you lose weight and feel more confident you will find people do stick with you and prefer you energetic and happy. You can also tell yourself you are doing a favour for your family—you'll be healthier, more positive and probably around longer.

So first you need to believe you can and want to do this for yourself. And then you need to practise saying no in situations that carry with them a sense of risk. It often helps to join the "no" with options. Here are some examples to help you get going.

Scenario 1. A friend urges you to have a piece of cake you don't want. After your first, "No, thank you," she moves to guilt: "Oh, come on. I know it's your favourite—that's why I got it."

Answer: "Thank you—it was very thoughtful of you but I'm trying to lose weight—let's plan to celebrate together with a piece of this cake when I reach my target weight."

It is worth noting that true friends will want you to succeed. Some people may be threatened by your success and work to undermine you. They are not true friends.

Scenario 2. Your partner says, "I don't like to eat desserts alone—so have a small piece with me."

Answer 1: "I can make green-light desserts in the future and we can share them."

Answer 2: "Hey, I need your help being successful so please don't tempt me."

Answer 3: "No, I'm not eating that dessert but let me get some fruit so I can keep you company."

Note that none of the answers is confrontational. It's always most comfortable for ESIs to avoid conflict.

ESIs also need to practise in some non-eating situations. Practise responding positively to comments about your weight loss and appearance. ESIs will usually slough off anything complimentary, assuming people don't really mean it or they are just trying to make the ESIs feel better. Try smiling and saying "Thank you" and looking the person in the eye. And practise saying no to doing things you don't want to do. Saying no to a social invitation that doesn't really tempt you does not mean you will hurt feelings or the person will cross you off his or her list and abandon the friendship.

Scenario 3. A friend calls and says "I'm going to the mall—do you want to come?" Answer: "Thanks for asking but I have other things I need to do."

Scenario 4. A friend suggests movie X.

Answer: "I wasn't planning to see that. Have you thought about movie Y?"

For each week of success on the diet, try to reward yourself with something personal that contributes to your sense of wellness and attractiveness, such as a manicure, a new haircut or a makeup makeover at the local department store.

Keep a diary or journal of your personal story. Record all the successes you have. Record experiences of asserting what you wanted, the feelings and the outcomes. Make special note that the outcomes were not catastrophic!

Grazing and eating without thinking is a temporary way of comfort for ESIs. Often ESIs experience little real pleasure when grazing and feel both helpless and hopeless when they do it. So stick a note on the fridge door: I will regret grazing—this is not what I want to do for myself. (If you are too self-conscious to actually post the note, then just keep those words in your mind when your hand is on the fridge door.) You can also use the tips provided for the IEs (see pages 77–81).

In summary:

- Recognize that we are our own harshest critics.
- Practise making choices you want and finding out the sky does not fall.
- Practise saying no when you don't want to do something.
- Practise accepting compliments and positive feedback.
- Eat foods you really enjoy.
- Keep a diary of your journey and responses.
- Reward successes.
- Keep reminding yourself—this is for me and I deserve it!.

GENERAL EATING BEHAVIOURS

Now that I have covered the basic personality traits and their associated eating behaviours, let's look at some general eating behaviours for which we are all at risk.

1. SKIPPING BREAKFAST

This is a very common bad habit. It is estimated that one-quarter of North Americans skip breakfast and the numbers are even worse for teenagers. A study of U.S. teens showed that only 32 percent eat breakfast regularly.

Breakfast is the most important meal of the day. By the time people get up in the morning, most haven't eaten for ten to twelve hours. Skipping breakfast will almost certainly result in snacking throughout the day to stave off hunger and flagging energy levels. And chances are that you will reach for high-calorie, high-fat foods such as doughnuts, muffins or cookies to give you that quick fix your body feels it needs. At the end of the day, chances are you'll be starving and unnecessarily stuffing yourself at dinner. None of these activities will help shrink your waistline—quite the reverse.

2. NOT TAKING TIME TO EAT PROPERLY

Saying "I don't have time to eat properly" creates a spawning ground for bad habits. People who don't take the time to eat properly tend to grab a coffee and Danish on their way to work;

eat a store-bought muffin mid-morning to boost flagging energy levels; have a slice or two of pizza with a soft drink for lunch; snack on chocolate and cookies in the afternoon in a desperate attempt to keep their eyes open; pick up some high-fat takeout food on the way home for dinner; and finally collapse in front of the TV for the evening with beer and a bowl of pretzels. Sound familiar?

It's easy to slip into this harmful cycle of fattening convenience food and short-term energy fixes, but you'll pay for the convenience with a growing girth and mood swings as your blood sugars rocket up and down. And really, the amount of time required to prepare your own healthy meals and snacks is quite modest. Fifteen minutes in the morning is all it takes to prepare and eat a healthy breakfast—often the length of time it takes to line up for a coffee. If you can't manage to wake up fifteen minutes earlier to squeeze in a nutritious breakfast before rushing off to work, then bring along a box of green-light cereal, a carton of skim milk and piece of fruit. A piece of fruit and carton of skim milk takes no time to prepare and makes a filling, nutritious snack. And there are always places you can get a green-light sandwich so you don't have to resort to pizza. Eating healthily through the day will ensure that you have the energy when you arrive home to prepare a quick green-light dinner in the time it would have taken to drive to the takeout place and wait for your order.

3. GRAZING

The world's best grazers are teenagers. They simply cannot avoid opening the fridge every time they pass it. Their rapid growth and (we hope) high activity levels require a constant high-calorie intake. Unfortunately, grazing is a habit that many people continue into their adult lives when this need for a high-calorie intake is past, with disastrous results for their waistlines and health. A few nuts here, a couple of cookies there, a tablespoon or two of peanut butter, and a few glasses of juice all look pretty harmless in themselves, but taken together, they can easily total several hundred extra calories a day! And those can add up to over twenty pounds of additional weight in a year.

On the G.I. Diet, you should be eating three meals plus three snacks a day, which means you are eating something approximately every two to three waking hours. This will reduce your temptation to graze. One reader wrote that she couldn't believe how she could be losing weight when she always seemed to be eating. She called it "green-light grazing"!

4. UNCONSCIOUS EATING

How often have you begun to nibble on a bowl of chips or nuts or a box of cookies while watching TV, reading a book or talking on the phone and then suddenly realized that you've eaten the whole lot? Too often, I would guess.

Eating should never be a peripheral activity—it should always be the focus. Eat your meals at the table, and set aside distractions such as the TV, computer, video game or telephone while you have your snacks. This will help you to always eat consciously and be aware of exactly how much you are eating.

5. EATING TOO QUICKLY

The famous Dr. Johnson of the eighteenth century is said to have asserted that food should always be chewed thirty-two times before swallowing. Though this seems rather excessive, there is some truth here. Many of us tend to eat far too quickly. It takes twenty to thirty minutes for the stomach to let the brain know it is full. If you eat too quickly, you'll continue to eat past the point at which you've had enough. The solution, then, is to eat slowly to allow the brain to catch up with your stomach.

That's probably another reason that Mediterranean countries have lower rates of obesity: they take far longer to eat their meals. In these countries, mealtimes are for family and friends, and for enjoying the pleasure of food—not simply a means to tackle hunger.

A recent investigation into the amount of time spent at meals around the world placed France as having the longest mealtimes and Canada as having virtually the shortest (second from the bottom). Needless to say, France has one of the lowest obesity rates in the Western world.

To ensure you are not eating more than your appetite requires, slow down and really enjoy what you are eating. Put your fork down between mouthfuls. Savour the flavour and textures.

6. NOT DRINKING ENOUGH

Did you know that by the time you feel thirsty you are already dehydrated? Your body's need for water is second only to its need for oxygen. Up to 70 percent of the body is water, and we should be drinking about eight glasses of fluids a day to replenish our supply. Yet many of us don't take the time to drink enough, and we go tired and hungry, which makes us reach for food when we really should be reaching for a glass of water. Our body isn't hungry, it's thirsty. So always carry water with you and make sure you are drinking the recommended amount. Being properly hydrated will go a long way toward helping you control your appetite and lose weight.

7. REWARDING FOR EXERCISE

Another common habit is to reward yourself with food for doing some exercise. Rather than allowing the reward to lie in the exercise itself, many people believe that the extra effort deserves some form of additional reward or treat, which more often than not takes the form of food or drink.

Unfortunately, a latte on the way home from the gym can more than offset your hard-earned calorie loss.

8. CLEANING THE PLATE

Many of us were taught from a young age to finish what's on our plates. This habit does not, unfortunately, help us in later life to lose or maintain weight. We not only finish our own plate, but also tend to finish the leftovers on our children's plates or that last lonely slice in the pie dish. I confess that I do this. But this habit causes us to eat more than we need to satisfy our hunger and is therefore dreadful for weight control. Get into the habit of letting your stomach and brain decide when you are full, not the quantity of food on your plate. Put out only enough food for the meal, no extras. Leftovers can always be stored in the fridge, rather than around your waist or hips.

9. SHOPPING ON AN EMPTY STOMACH

When you are full and satisfied, food shopping is rarely top of mind. But when you are hungry, grocery shopping suddenly seems like a very good idea indeed. Unfortunately, it just isn't: you'll end up with a shopping cart that has been filled primarily by your stomach rather than your head. Those red-light foods will seem far more tempting than usual, and you will probably make some poor choices as a result.

So always shop after a meal, or at least take a green-light snack such as a homemade muffin or a high protein bar with you. You'll make far wiser choices this way.

10. EATING HIGH-SUGAR, HIGH-FAT TREATS

As we are all only too aware, food is a big part of holidays and celebrations—just think of Thanksgiving, a wedding, a bar mitzvah or Christmas and you'll probably picture the special foods that go along with them. Where would the candy industry be without Valentine's Day, Halloween or Easter? Food is inextricably linked with positive experiences, and that is one of the reasons we often think of certain foods as "treats." Whether it's Grandma doling out candies to a child who has been good, or a neighbour presenting you with a freshly baked pie as a reward for raking her leaves, we are accustomed to using food treats to reward the people in our lives as well as ourselves. Unfortunately, these so-called treats tend to be high in calories, sugar and fat and are certainly not your friends. They are a major contributor to the obesity crisis and to weight-related diseases such as diabetes and heart disease. We should really start to view these foods as penalties rather than rewards.

Instead, choose treats that are lower in calories and fat. If candy is your thing, there is a plethora of low- and no-sugar brands available. Fresh fruit, low-fat, sugar-free yogurt and low-fat frozen yogurt are even better treats. And there are many delicious green-light dessert and snack recipes in all my G.I. Diet books. Treats are a wonderful part of our lives—just make sure they are the right sort of treats.

Keep in mind that while it will take some effort and can be challenging at times to change bad habits, it's well worthwhile to persevere with beneficial new behaviours. Before you know it, they'll be second nature; new habits as firmly entrenched as the old ones used to be. But these ones will help you slim down to a brand new you.

EMOTIONAL EATING

When we have reasonably balanced lives, food plays an important but not dominant role in our day-to-day life. We all eat for comfort. For example, when we are sick we may eat certain favourite foods that make us "feel better." Often these are foods from our childhood that we associate with being looked after. When things are out of balance and we don't feel good about certain aspects of our lives then food can take over. Eating can be a means for dealing with stressful situations. This can happen regardless of your particular personality traits so I recommend that everyone read this section even if there is some overlap in the content with the previous discussion of your particular personality traits.

Frequently, eating to feel better is preceded by negative feelings. For some people, it will be feelings of sadness, loneliness or even a sense of boredom. For others, the feelings can be more in the range of anger, irritability or high stress. These feelings can lead to a vicious food eating cycle. It goes something like this:

I feel: depressed; angry; bored; sad; bad about myself (low self-esteem) ➔ so I eat to feel better ➔ I experience a brief blood sugar high and feel better ➔ I experience a blood sugar crash and feel terrible ➔ I feel bad about myself for eating, for failing ➔ so I eat to feel better ... and around I go.

In many situations the original reasons for feeling bad about oneself, or getting angry, overwhelmed or disappointed, may have origins in childhood as I suggested in the section on the Eaters with Self-esteem Issues. Overeating, negative body image and low self-esteem are the consequences experienced by adults. Usually we do not make any conscious link between past events and current behaviour. For example, as a child, parental approval or love may have been connected with food via treats or eating everything served to us. Or we may have been punished (love withdrawn) if we didn't eat our vegetables! As a consequence, eating has become connected to trying to recapture that good feeling of being loved. Although we are not aware of these motives or psychological reasons for the behaviour, we have eaten for love or approval for so long that it has become part of our food and eating habits.

Rick's mother could not bear to see food unfinished regardless of whether or not a person was still hungry. Throughout her long life of 100 years she would say, "I do like to see a clean plate" when all the food on the table had disappeared. This attitude led to a learned behaviour on Rick's part that earned Rick, as a child, love and approval from his mother. As his wife, I learned to never put excess food on the table at mealtimes. One way I do this is to make up the dinner plates before I serve them—no self-service from large bowls—otherwise, Rick would unconsciously graze through a lot of extra food!

Just as I have recommended becoming aware of certain personality traits, if you want to change your emotional eating, you need to become aware of eating habits. For example, when you walk in the front door is the first stop the fridge or cookie cupboard? When you have had a bad day, do you deal with it by eating something sweet or creamy? When you feel bored and have nothing structured to do, is your first activity to eat? Are you unable to watch TV without food in your hand so that you end up unconsciously eating more than you realize? I help myself to a piece of dark chocolate most evenings if I am watching TV. One night I realized I was in the middle of eating a second piece with no memory of reaching down and picking it up! Henceforth, the chocolate bar stays in the fridge and I remove one piece for eating!

Review the eating habits we outlined on pages 77–81 earlier in this chapter. Take a day or two to jot down your habits and patterns and work out when automatic behaviours take over and when it is most difficult for you to avoid eating in excess. It is important to recognize risky situations. Consider if these eating habits intensify when you are stressed. Many women have told about the increased stress of trying to do it all—holding a full-time job while running a household, and raising a family and/or looking after aged parents. The first step is to consider alternative ways to cope, such as asking for help from others.

Once you are aware of how emotional eating plays a role in your life, you can begin to change your eating behaviour. You have already taken the first step by ensuring that all the food in your house and workplace, as well as all food going into your mouth, is green-light. Make sure you reward yourself for this accomplishment. Plan something nice: a book, a little something from the makeup counter, a trip to your favourite store (in Rick's case, Canadian Tire or Home Depot)—whatever ties into your interests or passions. Just make sure it isn't a red-light food!

Start by trying to modify one behaviour at a time. If you usually walk in the door and open the fridge, make sure something green-light is waiting for you there. The next week, try walking past the fridge and delaying the snack by thirty minutes or just take a few minutes for yourself—have a cup of tea and take a moment to breathe.

It is particularly important to have snacks with a good, sweet mouth feel when sugar cravings take over. Homemade green-light fruit muffins (use raspberries, blueberries, strawberries, peaches), make an excellent sweet snack as do fresh berries sweetened with Splenda and perhaps served with a dollop of Splenda-sweetened non-fat sour cream. Even sugar-free candies are better than that red-light chocolate bar. Sugar cravings and irritability will lessen as long as you stick with green-light foods and eat three meals and three snacks a day. Make up individual snacks in small bags so you always have snacks available. I carry small high-protein nutrition bars in my purse at all times so I can have half a bar snack available wherever I am.

Make a list of pleasurable activities you could be doing instead of eating. For example, if you sit in front of TV and eat, what else could you be doing with your hands? Many of us like to be doing something while watching TV; I read books or magazines. Some people do crafts or even get the ironing done! You can always turn off the TV—go for a walk, or use your e-reader and check out the bestseller lists. Finding pleasurable activities to substitute for eating helps to break the vicious cycle I described above.

It is very important to realize that as you lose weight, you will not only feel better physically but also feel better psychologically; being successful in this pursuit will improve your self-esteem. Feeling better about how you look is the best reinforcement for holding back on red-light foods, and breaking those bad eating habits. Not only will you notice your body changing but also others will notice. As you start to experience success in weight reduction—and we are talking here about permanent weight reduction—you start to experience the benefits of having accomplished a goal. People who have successfully lost weight often hold their bodies differently and interact with people in a more positive manner. Shoulders are less slumped and heads are held higher.

Let me stress again the need to find substitute activities. This is important for breaking those bad eating habits. Make a substitute activities list and use it until you feel sure that your new behaviours and eating patterns are your new habits. And don't beat up on yourself if you slip—it happens to all of us— just get back on the horse. Having the guts and determination to do this program takes courage so pat yourself on the back and get on with the journey.

I have been stressing immediate substitute activities but it may also be helpful to think about long-term goals. Have you always had a secret dream or goal? Maybe taking dance lessons, performing in a play or learning to ski? Perhaps you have avoided those dreams because of your self-esteem or body image. Maybe now is the time to recognize that this is something you could do. Keep that long-term goal in mind when you reach for that red-light food. How will that help you get to the dance floor?

A cardiologist friend of ours, who is struggling with some bad food habits and poor food choices, wears a plastic bracelet on his left wrist. When he makes a wrong choice, he switches the bracelet to his right wrist. This reminds him every time he reaches for something to eat that he has already made one poor choice that day already. He says it's worked for him, so if you want a visual aid to help remind you to break bad eating habits, then you might want to try this idea. Another reader determined that the weight she needed to lose was equal to the total weight of her two small children combined. Every time she felt tempted she picked up both her children and tried to walk briskly—an exhausting activity! It certainly helped her keep away from the red-light treats.

Finally, I encourage you to build in a reward for each week of success on the program—go to a show or a ball game, buy some flowers or have a long, scented bath. Don't buy the new wardrobe yet—that is for later. Just remember, be good to yourself.

—Dr. Ruth Gallop

Chapter Eight Cooking the Green-Light Way

EQUIPMENT

The right equipment will help you gain maximum nutritional benefit as well as save you time. Every G.I. Diet kitchen should have the following:

MICROWAVE OVEN

Heating and cooking foods is really the first step in the digestive process. The longer you cook your food, the more "digestible" it becomes. Ever tried eating a raw potato? It takes a week to digest! As a result, cooking raises the G.I. of foods because it replicates, in effect, what your digestive system would be doing. Remember, it's important to have your stomach doing as much of the processing as possible. Though we don't recommend always eating uncooked foods, we do suggest keeping cooking times minimal, or cooking only until, as the Italians say, *al dente* or "with some firmness to the bite."

One of the best ways of doing this is with a microwave oven. Fresh or frozen vegetables can be cooked in minutes, keeping the G.I. low and preserving nutrients better than other methods because cooking time is reduced and little or no water is used.

The microwave is also your best green-light kitchen friend for thawing meats and warming snacks or leftovers.

NONSTICK FRYING PANS

You should have two different sizes plus lids. They require little or no oil, and cleanup is a cinch. We are big on stir-fries in our household, so these nonstick skillets get a lot of use.

BARBECUES/INDOOR GRILLS

Cooking meat and fish on either a barbecue or indoor grill is a good idea as extra fat drains off—and the food always seems to taste better, too.

CONVERTING RECIPES

It's easy to make many of your own standby recipes green-light by following the guidelines below; you don't have to necessarily use the recipes listed in this book.

GREEN-LIGHT INGREDIENTS

First, ensure that all the ingredients in the recipe are green-light. If there are any red- or yellow-light ingredients, either omit or replace them with the green-light alternative. Some flavour enhancing red- and yellow-light foods can be used in recipes in very limited quantities, such as half a cup of wine in a dish that will serve six people, or 1/4 cup raisins in a salad for four. Full-flavoured cheeses can also be used sparingly. For example, a tablespoon or two of grated Parmesan cheese sprinkled over a casserole will add flavour without too many calories.

FIBRE

The fibre content of the recipe is critical. Fibre, both soluble and insoluble, is key to the overall G.I. rating of the recipe. The more the better. If your recipe is light on fibre, consider adding fibre boosters such as oats, bran, whole grains or beans.

FAT

Recipes should be low in fat with little or no saturated fat. If oil is called for, use vegetable oil. Canola and olive oil are your best choices. Use as little as possible, as all fats are calorie-dense.

SUGAR

Never add sugar or sugar-based ingredients such as corn syrup or molasses. There are some excellent sugar substitutes available; our favourite is Splenda, which was developed from a sugar base but does not have the calories. Splenda works well in cooking and baking. Measure it by volume (not weight) to effectively replace sugar. For example, 1 tablespoon sugar equals 1 tablespoon Splenda. Note that Brown Splenda is 50 percent sugar and is therefore not recommended. Sugar Twin Brown is an acceptable alternative.

PROTEIN

Be sure that your recipe contains sufficient protein, or that you are serving it alongside some protein to round out the meal. Protein helps slow the digestive process, which effectively lowers the G.I. of a recipe. It is also the one component that is often overlooked at mealtime, particularly in recipes for salads and snacks. Useful protein boosters include low-fat dairy products; lean meats, poultry and seafood; egg whites; beans; and soy-based foods, such as soy or whey powders.

FOOD PREPARATION BASICS

MEAT

Pork loin, top or eye round beef, veal and lean deli ham are your best choices. Red meat in general is a yellow-light food, although for pragmatic reasons I've included lean cuts of beef and extra-lean ground beef in Phase I. Most cuts of pork and lamb tend to have a higher fat content and should be avoided until Phase II. Serving size is critical. Remember: use the palm of your hand or a pack of playing cards as a guide to portion size. Do not be alarmed by the modest size of these portions. I had a real problem downsizing my steak at first, but now my stomach rebels at the portions served in many restaurants.

Steak: Basic Preparation

Per person

1. Broil or barbecue a fully trimmed top or eye round steak (4 ounces per person).

2. Sauté sliced onions and mushrooms with a little water in a nonstick skillet, and serve with steak.

3. Season chopped broccoli, asparagus, and halved Brussels sprouts with nutmeg and pepper, then microwave on high power until tender, 3 to 5 minutes.

4. Boil 3 tablespoons uncooked basmati rice, or two to three small new potatoes, per person. Season the cooked potatoes with herbs and a touch of olive oil.

Poultry: Basic Preparation

1 serving

Naturally low in fat, cooked chicken or turkey breast can be prepared in dozens of ways, and combined with a variety of herbs, spices and vegetables to enhance its flavour.

Vegetable oil cooking spray (preferably canola or olive oil)
4 oz skinless, boneless chicken breast or turkey breast, whole, sliced, or cubed

1. Spray oil in a small nonstick skillet, and then place it over medium-high heat.

2. Add the chicken or turkey breast and sauté until firm to the touch and no longer pink, about 4 minutes per side for 1 chicken breast or piece of turkey, or 5 to 6 minutes for slices or cubes.

Fish: Basic Preparation

1 serving

Virtually any fish is suitable, but never use commercially breaded or battered versions. Salmon and trout are favourites in our house. Prespiced or flavoured fish varieties are okay, but why pay someone else a whopping premium for what you can easily do yourself?

Here are directions for cooking fish fillets in a microwave oven. It couldn't be easier. Proportions can be multiplied as necessary.

1 fish fillet (4 oz)
1–2 tsp fresh lemon juice
Black pepper

1. Place the fish fillet in a microwave-safe dish.

2. Sprinkle the lemon juice and a dash of pepper over the fish.

3. Cover the dish with microwave-safe plastic wrap, folding back one corner slightly to allow the steam to escape.

4. Microwave the fish on high power until it is opaque and flakes when a fork is inserted, 4 to 5 minutes. Let stand for 2 minutes, then serve.

Variations

Sprinkle fish with fresh or dried herbs, such as dill, parsley, basil or tarragon.

Cook fish on a bed of leeks and onions. (Do not add oil.)

Sprinkle the fish with a mixture of whole wheat bread crumbs and chopped parsley (1 tablespoon per fillet) plus 1 teaspoon of melted light non-hydrogenated margarine.

Green-Light Side Dishes

Need some ideas for what to serve alongside poultry, fish or meat? Here are a few easy-to-prepare side dishes that will fit right in with the G.I. Diet.

- Green beans with almonds or mushrooms.
- Mixed vegetables, such as sliced carrots, broccoli or cauliflower florets, and halved Brussels sprouts.
- Boiled small, preferably new, potatoes (2 to 3 per serving), tossed with herbs and a smidgen of olive oil.
- Basmati rice (you can stir some extra vegetables into the rice during the last minute of cooking). Limit serving size to 3 tablespoons uncooked rice, which will give you 2/3 of a cup when cooked, covering one-quarter of the plate.
- Pasta—35 grams, uncooked, or 3/4 cup cooked, covering one-quarter of the plate.

Chapter Nine
Recipes

BREAKFAST

Oatmeal can be endlessly varied by changing the flavour of the fruit yogurt you add or by mixing in sliced fruit or berries. My wife's favourite way to eat oatmeal is with skim milk, unsweetened applesauce, sliced almonds and sweetener. Along with my oatmeal I like to have an orange and a glass of skim milk. It's a delicious breakfast that will stay with you all morning.

Oatmeal

1 serving
1/2 cup old-fashioned rolled oats
1 cup water or skim milk
1/2–3/4 cup nonfat fruit yogurt with sugar substitute
2 tbsp sliced almonds
Fresh or frozen berries

Place the oats in a microwave-safe bowl and cover with water or skim milk. Microwave the oats on medium power for 3 minutes. Mix in the yogurt, almonds and some fresh fruit.

Homemade Muesli

This is a delicious cold version of the oatmeal recipe.

2 servings
1 cup old-fashioned rolled oats
3/4 cup skim milk
3/4 cup nonfat fruit yogurt with sugar substitute
2 tbsp sliced almonds
3/4 cup diced apple or pear, or berries
Sweetener

Place the oats in a bowl, cover them with the milk, and let soak in the refrigerator overnight. Add the yogurt, almonds, fruit, and sweetener to taste, and mix well.

Basic Omelette and Variations

1 serving

Omelettes are easy to make and you can vary them by adding any number of fresh vegetables, a little cheese and/or some meat. You'll find ingredients for a basic omelette here, along with suggestions for making Italian, Mexican, vegetarian and Western versions. Don't stop with these—using the proportions as a guide, you can add whatever green-light ingredients strike your fancy. To round out the meal, include a cup of fresh fruit and a glass of skim milk or 1/2 to 3/4 cup of nonfat fruit yogurt with sugar substitute.

Vegetable oil cooking spray (preferably canola or olive oil)
1/2 cup liquid egg
1/4 cup skim milk

Italian Omelette
1/2 cup sliced mushrooms
1 oz grated skim mozzarella cheese
1/2 cup tomato purée
Chopped fresh or dried herbs, such as oregano or basil

Mexican Omelette
1 cup chopped red and green bell pepper
1/2 cup sliced mushrooms
1/2 cup canned beans, drained and rinsed
Hot sauce or chili powder (optional), for sprinkling over the omelette

Vegetarian Omelette
1 cup broccoli florets
1/2 cup sliced mushrooms
1/2 cup chopped red and green bell pepper
1 oz grated skim-milk cheese

Western Omelette
1 cup chopped red and green bell pepper
1 small onion, chopped
2 slices back bacon, lean deli ham or turkey breast
Chopped red pepper flakes or cayenne pepper (optional) for
  sprinkling over the omelette

Omelette Preparation

1. Spray oil in a small nonstick skillet, then place it over
medium heat.

2. Add the vegetables (variety depends on which omelette you
are making), and sauté until tender, about 5 minutes. Transfer
the vegetables to a plate and cover with aluminum foil to keep
warm.

3. Beat the eggs with the milk and pour them into the skillet
over medium heat. Cook until the eggs start to firm up, then
spread the warm vegetables, cheese, herbs, beans, and/or
meat over them. Continue cooking until the eggs are done to
your liking.

4. If desired, sprinkle the omelette with hot sauce, chili powder,
red pepper flakes or cayenne, then serve.

*Variation: Make scrambled eggs by stirring the eggs as they cook,
and adding any additional ingredients while the eggs are still soft.*

Huevos Rancheros

These eggs are a spicy way to start the day and are very filling.
They are poached to perfection in the oven, so you can enjoy
your guests while brunch cooks away.

2 tsp canola oil
1 onion, chopped
2 cloves garlic, minced
1 small jalapeño pepper, minced
1 tbsp chili powder
1 tsp dried oregano
1 tsp ground cumin

1 can (398 mL) stewed tomatoes
1 cup vegetable cocktail or tomato juice
1 can (540 mL) black beans, drained and rinsed
1 can (540 mL) chickpeas, drained and rinsed
1 green bell pepper, finely chopped
1/4 cup chopped fresh cilantro
2 tbsp chopped fresh flat-leaf parsley
6 eggs
6 small whole wheat tortillas

1. Heat the oil over medium heat in a large nonstick skillet and cook the onion, garlic, jalapeño pepper, chili powder, oregano and cumin until the onion starts to soften, about 3 minutes. Add the tomatoes, vegetable juice, black beans, chickpeas, green pepper, and half each of the cilantro and parsley, and bring to a boil. Reduce the heat and simmer until slightly thickened, about 15 minutes. Pour the mixture into a 9 × 13-inch baking dish.

2. Preheat the oven to 425°F.

3. Break 1 egg into a small bowl and carefully slide it onto the bean mixture. Repeat with the remaining eggs, spacing them out like cookies on a baking sheet. Cover the dish with aluminum foil and bake until the whites of the eggs are set (or longer if desired), about 10 minutes. Sprinkle the remaining cilantro and parsley over the dish and serve with tortillas.

Makes 6 servings.

Southwest Omelette Roll-Up

Brunch is a great time to gather with friends and family, but you don't want to spend all your time at the stove. Here is a family-sized omelette with a southwest bean filling that you can make ahead of time. It's perfect with a salad and fresh fruit.

Roux:
2 tbsp canola oil
3 tbsp whole wheat flour
1 cup warm skim milk
1/4 tsp salt
Pinch of black pepper
Pinch of ground cumin (optional)

Omelette:
4 egg whites
1 cup liquid egg

Filling:
1 package (250 g) light cream cheese, softened
1/2 cup low-fat salsa
1 can (540 mL) red kidney beans or black beans, drained and
   rinsed
1 red or green bell pepper, diced
2 green onions, sliced
1/4 cup chopped fresh cilantro or flat-leaf parsley

1. **Make the roux:** Heat the oil in a small saucepan over medium heat and add the flour. Cook for 1 minute, whisking constantly. Slowly add the milk and cook, whisking gently, until thick enough to coat the back of a spoon, about 5 minutes. Whisk in the salt, pepper and cumin, if using, and whisk to combine thoroughly. Pour into a large bowl and let cool.

2. Preheat the oven to 350°F. Grease an 11 × 17-inch baking sheet and line it with parchment paper.

3. **Make the omelette:** Meanwhile, in another bowl, beat the egg whites to stiff peaks. Whisk the liquid egg into the roux and fold half of the egg whites into the mixture. Add the remaining egg whites, folding gently until combined. Pour the mixture onto the prepared baking sheet.

4. Bake until the eggs are puffed, lightly golden, and firm to the touch, about 18 minutes. Let cool on the baking sheet.

5. **Make the filling:** Combine the cream cheese and salsa in a large bowl and stir until smooth. Stir in the beans, red pepper, green onions and cilantro and set aside.

6. Run a small knife around the edges of the baking sheet and place a clean tea towel over the top. Invert the eggs onto a work surface and gently peel off the parchment paper. Spread the filling evenly over the eggs, leaving a 2-inch border on one of the long sides.

7. Using the tea towel as a guide, roll up the omelette starting with the other long side and working toward the long side with the 2-inch border. Cut in half to make 2 rolls. Using a long

spatula or palette knife, transfer the rolls to a large serving platter. Cut each roll into 4 pieces before serving.

Makes 8 servings.

Green Eggs and Ham

A beloved childhood story comes to life, with very healthy results. Spinach adds colour and flavour to the egg mixture, and lean ham adds a salty zing. This is a recipe that begs to be shared with family and friends at a festive breakfast.

1 tsp canola oil
1 small onion, finely diced
1 clove garlic, minced
2 red bell peppers, thinly sliced
1/4 cup chopped fresh flatleaf parsley
1/4 tsp dried basil or marjoram, or 1 tsp chopped fresh
1 tbsp Dijon mustard
6 slices lean ham or back bacon

Green Eggs:
1 bag (300 g) baby spinach
1 tsp canola oil
2 cups liquid egg
1/2 tsp salt
1/4 tsp black pepper
2 tbsp chopped fresh flat-leaf parsley
2 tbsp chopped fresh basil

1. Heat the oil in a nonstick skillet over medium heat. Add the onion and garlic and cook for 3 minutes. Add the peppers, parsley and basil and cook until the peppers are tendercrisp, about 3 minutes. Scrape the mixture into a 9 × 13-inch baking dish.

2. Spread each ham slice with some of the mustard and place the slices on top of the pepper mixture in a layer. Set aside.

3. Make the Green Eggs: Rinse the spinach in a colander and let drain. Heat a large nonstick skillet over medium-high heat. Add the spinach, in batches if necessary; cover; and cook until bright green and wilted, about 3 minutes. Drain again, let cool somewhat, and squeeze any excess water out. Chop the spinach and set it aside.

4. Preheat the oven to 400°F.

5. Heat the oil in a nonstick skillet over medium heat. Meanwhile, whisk together in a large bowl the liquid egg, salt and pepper. Add the chopped spinach and stir to combine.

6. Pour the spinach-egg mixture into the skillet and cook, without stirring, until the mixture begins to set around the edges. Lift one of the edges with a spatula and

7. Tilt the pan so the uncooked portion flows underneath. Sprinkle the parsley and basil over the eggs and continue cooking until the eggs are just set.

8. Cut the eggs into six portions and spoon one portion of the cooked eggs onto each of the ham slices. Cover the dish with aluminum foil and bake for about 10 minutes to warm through.

Makes 6 servings.

SOUPS

Cream of Spinach Soup

Many creamed soups contain, as their names suggest, cream. Some others get a creamy texture from the addition of puréed potatoes. This soup calls for puréed white kidney beans, which add fibre, flavour and creaminess while keeping it green-light.

1 tsp canola oil
1 onion, chopped
1 stalk celery, chopped
1 carrot, chopped
2 cloves garlic, minced
1 tbsp chopped fresh thyme, or 1 tsp dried
2 tomatoes, chopped
5 cups vegetable or chicken broth (low-fat, low-sodium)
1 can (540 mL) white kidney beans, drained and rinsed
1 bag (300 g) baby spinach, trimmed
Pinch each of salt and black pepper

1. Heat the oil in a soup pot over medium heat. Add the onion, celery, carrot, garlic and thyme and cook until the onion has softened, about 5 minutes. Add the tomatoes and cook for 2 minutes. Add the vegetable broth and beans and bring to a boil. Reduce the heat and simmer for 10 minutes.

2. Meanwhile, using a chef's knife, finely chop the spinach, then set it aside.

3. Working in batches, purée the soup in a blender until smooth, then return the soup to the pot. Bring to a gentle boil and add the spinach, salt and pepper. Cook, stirring, until the spinach is tender, wilted and bright green, about 5 minutes.

Makes 4 to 6 servings.

Cauliflower and Chickpea Soup

This combination will help you find another reason to buy cauliflower again—it's absolutely delicious with a hint of ginger and cumin.

1 tsp canola oil
1 onion, peeled and chopped
2 cloves garlic, minced
1 each carrot and celery stalk, chopped
1 tbsp minced peeled ginger
2 tsp ground cumin
1/2 tsp ground coriander
1/4 tsp ground turmeric
6 cups chopped cauliflower
2 cans (540 mL each) chickpeas, drained and rinsed
6 cups vegetable or chicken broth (low-fat, low-sodium)
1/2 cup nonfat plain yogurt
3 tbsp chopped fresh cilantro

1. Heat the oil in a soup pot over medium heat. Add the onion, garlic, carrot, celery, ginger, cumin, coriander and turmeric and cook until the onion has softened, about 5 minutes. Add the cauliflower and chickpeas and cook, stirring, about 2 minutes. Add the vegetable broth and bring to a boil. Cover, and simmer until the cauliflower is tender, about 20 minutes.

2. Transfer the soup to a blender or food processor and, working in batches, purée until smooth. Return the soup to the pot and reheat. Serve with a dollop of yogurt and a sprinkle of cilantro.

Makes 6 to 8 servings.

Storage: Once the soup is completely cool you can store it in airtight containers in the refrigerator for up to 3 days, or freeze it for up to 1 month.

Note: You will need to buy 1 small head of cauliflower (about 2 pounds) to get 6 cups of chopped cauliflower.

Southwest Chicken and Bean Soup

This has the flavour of a chicken chili but the consistency of a soup. You can make your own nacho chips to serve alongside by cutting whole wheat pitas into 8 wedges each and toasting them on a baking sheet in a 400°F oven for 10 minutes.

1 tsp canola oil
1 onion, finely chopped
2 cloves garlic, minced
2 tsp chili powder
1/2 tsp paprika
1/2 tsp ground cumin
6 cups chicken broth (low-fat, low-sodium)
1 can (398 mL) stewed tomatoes
1 each red and green bell pepper, diced
12 oz boneless chicken, finely chopped
1 can (425 g) red kidney beans, drained and rinsed
2 tbsp chopped fresh cilantro
2 tbsp fresh lime juice

1. Heat the oil in a soup pot over medium heat. Add the onion, garlic, chili powder, paprika and cumin and cook until the onion has softened, about 5 minutes.

2. Add the chicken broth, tomatoes and red and green peppers, and bring to a boil. Reduce the heat to a gentle boil and add the chicken and beans. Cook, stirring, for about 8 minutes or until the chicken is no longer pink inside. Add the cilantro and lime juice before serving.

Makes 4 servings.

SALADS

Here are five easy-to-prepare lunchtime salads:

Mixed Bean Salad

2 servings
1 can (540 mL) mixed beans, drained and rinsed
1/2 cucumber, chopped
1 tomato, chopped
1 cup cooked whole wheat pasta (small shells, macaroni or
  similar shape)
2 tbsp chopped fresh flat-leaf parsley
1 tbsp red wine vinegar
2 tsp olive oil
1/4 tsp Dijon mustard
Pinch each of salt and black pepper
Pinch of dried herbs, such as thyme or oregano

1. Place beans in large bowl and add cucumber, tomato, pasta
and parsley.

2. In small bowl, whisk together vinegar, oil, mustard, salt,
pepper and thyme. Pour over salad and toss to coat.

Greek Salad

2 servings
2 cups torn iceberg lettuce
1/2 cucumber, chopped
2 tomatoes, chopped
6 kalamata olives
1/2 red onion, sliced
1/4 cup crumbled feta
1 tbsp red wine vinegar
2 tsp extra-virgin olive oil
1 tsp fresh lemon juice
1/4 tsp dried oregano
Pinch each of salt and black pepper

1. In bowl, toss together lettuce, cucumber, tomatoes, red onion, olives and crumbled feta.

2. In small bowl, whisk together vinegar, oil, lemon juice, oregano and salt and pepper. Pour dressing over greens and toss.

Waldorf Chicken and Rice Salad

1 serving
3/4 cup cooked basmati or brown rice
1 medium apple, chopped
1 or 2 stalks celery, chopped
1/4 cup walnuts
4 oz cooked chicken, chopped
1 tbsp store-bought light buttermilk dressing

Place the rice, apple, celery, walnuts and chicken in a bowl. Pour the buttermilk dressing over and stir to mix. Refrigerate until serving time.

Basic Pasta Salad

1 serving
1/2–3/4 cup cooked whole wheat pasta (spirals, shells or similar shape)
1 cup chopped cooked vegetables (such as broccoli, asparagus, bell peppers or green onions)
1/4 cup light tomato sauce or other low-fat or nonfat pasta sauce
4 oz chopped cooked chicken or other lean meat, such as ground lean turkey or lean chicken sausage

Place the pasta, vegetables, tomato sauce and chicken in a bowl and stir to mix well. Refrigerate the salad, covered, until serving time, then heat it in the microwave or serve chilled.

Variation: You can use the proportions here as a guide and vary the vegetables, sauce and source of protein to suit your taste and add variety to your pasta salad lunches.

Cottage Cheese and Fruit

1 serving
Perfect for a lunch on the run.

1 cup low-fat cottage cheese
1 cup chopped fresh fruit or fruit canned in juice, such as
  peaches, apricots or pears

Place the cottage cheese and fruit in a plastic bowl with a
fitted lid, and stir to mix. Refrigerate until lunchtime.

*Variation: Replace the chopped fruit with a tablespoon of
double-fruit, low-sugar preserves.*

Mediterranean Rice Salad with Tangy
Mustard Herb Dressing

Here's a great dinner, and the leftovers (if there are any) are
just as good the next day for lunch. Meat lovers can feel free
to add sliced ham or turkey.

1 1/2 cups vegetable or chicken broth
3/4 cup brown rice
1/4 tsp salt
2 cups lightly packed baby spinach leaves
2 cups shredded red-leaf lettuce
2 tomatoes, chopped
1 can (540 mL) mixed beans, drained and rinsed
1 zucchini, diced
1 red bell pepper, diced
1 cup diced cucumber
2 hard-boiled eggs, peeled and quartered

Tangy Mustard Herb Dressing:
1/4 cup rice vinegar
2 tbsp chopped fresh basil
2 tbsp chopped fresh flat-leaf parsley
1 tbsp extra-virgin olive oil
2 tsp Dijon mustard
1/4 tsp each salt and black pepper

1. Bring the broth, rice and salt to a boil in a soup pot. Reduce the heat to low, cover, and cook until the liquid is absorbed, about 35 minutes. Remove from the heat and let stand for about 5 minutes. Fluff the rice with a fork and let cool slightly.

2. Meanwhile, put the spinach, lettuce, tomatoes, beans, zucchini, red pepper and cucumber in a large serving bowl. Add the rice and toss to combine. Scatter the egg on top.

3. **Make the Tangy Mustard Herb Dressing:** Whisk together in a small bowl the vinegar, basil, parsley, oil, mustard, salt and pepper.

4. Pour over the salad and toss gently to coat.

Makes 4 to 6 servings.

Niçoise Salad

Here's a salad that is a meal in itself. You can enjoy fresh grilled tuna instead of canned when available. Look for firm, bright-coloured tuna that has no fishy aroma. Grill for about 2 minutes per side for a perfect rare tuna steak.

1 lb green beans, trimmed
2 cups torn red-leaf lettuce
2 cups torn Boston lettuce
4 small new potatoes, cooked
2 cans (170 g each) chunk white tuna, drained
2 hard-boiled eggs
1 can (540 mL) chickpeas, drained and rinsed
1 cup grape tomatoes
1/2 small red onion, thinly sliced (optional)
1/4 cup small pitted black olives

Anchovy Mustard Vinaigrette:
1 anchovy fillet, minced, or 1 tsp anchovy paste
1 tbsp Dijon mustard
1 small clove garlic, minced
1/4 cup white wine vinegar
2 tbsp extra-virgin olive oil
1/4 tsp salt
1/4 tsp black pepper

Pinch of paprika
2 tbsp chopped fresh basil or flat-leaf parsley

1. Bring a saucepan of water to a boil. Add the green beans and cook until tender-crisp, about 7 minutes. Drain them, and rinse under cold water until cool. Set aside.

2. Spread the red-leaf and Boston lettuce onto a large platter. Cut the potatoes in quarters and arrange them attractively on the lettuce. Add the cooked beans, tuna, eggs, chickpeas, tomatoes, red onion, if using, and olives.

3. Make the Anchovy Mustard Vinaigrette: In a bowl, mash the anchovy fillet with a fork and add the Dijon mustard and garlic. Continue to mash to combine. Whisk in the vinegar, oil, salt, pepper and paprika. Drizzle the vinaigrette over the salad platter. Sprinkle with the basil.

Makes 4 to 6 servings.

Jerk Pork Salad

Jerk is a traditional Jamaican seasoning used to spice up pork, chicken and fish. Hot peppers give this some bite, and herbs lend flavour that has a cooling effect.

3 green onions, chopped
1 large clove garlic, chopped
1/2 each green and red bell pepper, chopped
1 small scotch bonnet or jalapeño pepper, seeded
1 tbsp chopped fresh thyme or 1 tsp dried
1 tsp each ground allspice and nutmeg
1/2 tsp black pepper
2 tbsp fresh lime juice
1 tbsp canola oil
2 pork tenderloins (12 oz each)
Chili Lime Vinaigrette:
2 tbsp apple cider vinegar
2 tsp each Dijon mustard and canola oil
1/2 tsp grated lime zest
1 tbsp fresh lime juice
1/2 tsp sugar substitute
1/4 tsp chili powder

Pinch each of salt and black pepper
6 cups mixed baby greens
1 cup halved grape tomatoes
1 cup chopped cucumber
1 can (540 mL) mixed beans, drained and rinsed

1. Preheat an outdoor grill or a grill pan.

2. Combine in a food processor the green onions, garlic, green
and red bell peppers, scotch bonnet pepper, thyme, allspice,
nutmeg and black pepper. Pulse until a smooth paste forms.
Pulse in the lime juice and oil.

3. Place the tenderloins in a shallow dish and spread with the
jerk seasoning, turning to coat. Cover and refrigerate for at
least 20 minutes and up to 8 hours.

4. **Make the Chili Lime Vinaigrette:** Whisk together in a small
bowl the vinegar, mustard, oil, lime zest and juice, sugar
substitute, chili powder, salt and black pepper.

5. Place the tenderloins on the greased grill over medium-high
heat. Cook, turning occasionally, for about 20 minutes or until
only a hint of pink remains. Remove to a plate.

6. In a serving bowl, toss together the baby greens, tomatoes,
cucumber and mixed beans. Pour the vinaigrette over the salad
and toss to coat.

7. Thinly slice the pork tenderloins and serve on top of the
greens.

Makes 6 servings.

Shrimp Caesar Salad

Caesar salad is wonderful as a meal, and by adding grilled chicken
breast or roasted salmon fillet you can change the flavour.
3 slices whole wheat bread
2 tbsp finely chopped fresh flat-leaf parsley
2 cloves garlic, minced
2 tsp extra-virgin olive oil
1/2 tsp dried basil
Pinch each of salt and black pepper
4 cups chopped romaine lettuce

1 can (540 mL) mixed beans, drained and rinsed
1 cup grape tomatoes, halved
12 oz large cooked shrimp

Anchovy Garlic Dressing:
3 cloves garlic, minced
2 anchovy fillets, finely minced (see Helpful Hint)
2 tsp Dijon mustard
3 tbsp chicken broth (low-fat, low-sodium)
4 tsp extra-virgin olive oil
1 tbsp fresh lemon juice
1/4 tsp each salt and black pepper

1. Preheat the oven to 400°F.

2. Cut the bread into 6-inch pieces and place them in a bowl. Add the parsley, garlic, oil, basil, salt and pepper and toss to coat well. Spread the bread onto a baking sheet lined with parchment paper and bake until golden and crisp, about 15 minutes. Let cool.

3. In a large serving bowl, combine the lettuce, beans, tomatoes and shrimp. Set aside.

4. **Make the Anchovy Garlic Dressing:** In a small bowl, mash together with a fork the garlic, anchovies and mustard. Whisk in the chicken broth, oil, lemon juice, salt and pepper.

5. Pour the dressing over the salad and toss to coat. Sprinkle with croutons before serving.

Makes 4 servings.

Helpful Hint: You can use 2 tsp anchovy paste instead of the anchovy fillets. Look for it in the dairy section.

MEATLESS

Vegetarian Shepherd's Pie

Here is a lighter twist on a traditionally quite heavy dish.
While a traditional shepherd's pie is filled with ground beef or
lamb, this one is filled instead with bulgur and beans. It's still
comforting and filled with protein, just healthier. Bulgur is also
sold as "Middle Eastern pasta" or cracked wheat. If you like, you
can skip the potato topping and serve the pie in bowls, like chili.

1 tsp canola oil
1 small onion, finely chopped
2 cloves garlic, minced
3/4 cup bulgur
1 tsp dried oregano
1/2 tsp dried basil
1 1/2 cups vegetable broth
1 cup canned stewed tomatoes with juices
2 new red potatoes
1/4 cup water
1 can (540 mL) chickpeas, drained and rinsed
1 cup frozen peas
1/2 tsp salt
1/2 tsp black pepper
2 tbsp chopped fresh flat-leaf parsley

1. Heat the oil in a nonstick skillet over medium heat. Add the
onion, garlic, bulgur, oregano and basil and cook until the onion
is softened, about 5 minutes. Add the broth and tomatoes,
breaking up the tomatoes with the back of a spoon, and bring
to a boil. Reduce the heat to simmer, cover, and cook until the
bulgur is just tender, about 10 minutes.

2. Preheat the oven to 400°F.

3. Meanwhile, pierce the potatoes all over with a fork. Place
the potatoes in a small bowl with the water and microwave on
high for 5 minutes. Let cool.

4. Add the chickpeas, peas and half each of the salt and pepper
to the bulgur mixture and stir to combine. Scrape into an
8-inch casserole dish, smoothing the top.

5. Thinly slice the potatoes and layer them, overlapping slightly, on top of the bulgur mixture. Sprinkle with the remaining salt and pepper and the parsley.

6. Bake until the mixture is bubbly, about 20 minutes. Let cool slightly before serving.

Makes 4 servings.

Helpful Hint: If you prefer not to microwave the potatoes, boil them in a saucepan filled with enough water to cover them for about 10 minutes, or until tender but firm.

Bean and Onion Pizza

Here's a restaurant favourite that is custom-made for your G.I. lifestyle.

Pizza Dough:
3/4 cup warm water
2 1/4 tsp active dry yeast
1 1/3 cups whole wheat flour
1/2 cup wheat bran
Pinch of salt

Topping:
1 tsp canola oil
2 onions, thinly sliced
2 cloves garlic, minced
1/4 tsp dried thyme
Pinch each of salt and black pepper
1/4 cup sun-dried tomatoes
1/2 cup boiling water
1 cup cooked red kidney beans
3/4 cup low-fat pasta sauce
2 tbsp chopped fresh basil
3/4 cup crumbled light feta cheese

1. Make the Pizza Dough: Pour the water into a large bowl and sprinkle with the yeast. Let stand for about 10 minutes or until frothy. Stir in 1 1/4 cups of the flour, the bran and salt until a ragged dough forms. Let stand, covered, for 30 minutes. Place the dough onto a floured surface and knead it, adding more of the remaining flour as necessary, just until it forms a soft, slightly sticky dough. Place in a greased bowl, cover, and let rest until doubled in bulk, about 1 hour.

2. Make the Topping: Heat the oil in a nonstick skillet over medium-high heat. Add the onions and garlic and cook, stirring, until the onions are starting to become golden, about 3 minutes. Reduce the heat to medium and add the thyme, salt and pepper. Continue cooking, stirring occasionally, until the onions are soft and golden brown, about 15 minutes.

3. Soak the sun-dried tomatoes in the boiling water and let stand for 5 minutes. Drain and discard the water and chop the tomatoes.

4. Preheat the oven to 425°F. Punch down the dough and roll it out on a floured surface to fit a 12- to 14-inch round pizza pan. Place the dough on the pan, stretching it as necessary to fit.

5. Put the beans in a large mixing bowl and mash them with a potato masher. Stir in the pasta sauce, sun-dried tomatoes and basil. Spread the topping over the pizza dough. Top with the onions and sprinkle with feta.

6. Bake for about 20 minutes or until golden and crisp.

Makes 4 servings.

Mushroom and Bean Ragout

A ragout is a thick sauce that is wonderful served over noodles or rice. I like it served over radiatore or rotini pasta. You can also serve it on its own, like chili.

2 tsp extra-virgin olive oil
1 lb mushrooms, finely chopped
1 onion, chopped
4 cloves garlic, minced
1 small stalk celery, chopped
1 small carrot, diced
1 tsp each Italian herb seasoning and paprika
1 can (796 mL) diced tomatoes
1 can (540 mL) kidney beans, drained and rinsed
1/4 cup tomato paste
Pinch each of salt and black pepper

1. Heat the oil in a large, shallow Dutch oven over medium-high heat. Cook the mushrooms, onion, garlic, celery, carrot, Italian herb seasoning and paprika until the onion is golden and the liquid from the mushrooms evaporates, about 10 minutes.

2. Add the tomatoes, beans, tomato paste, salt and pepper and bring to a boil. Reduce the heat and simmer gently for about 25 minutes or until thickened.

Makes 4 servings.

White Bean Mash

This creamy side dish is a higher-fibre alternative to mashed potatoes. The creaminess comes from the addition of vegetable broth. Add your favourite greens like watercress for a peppery bite or kale for a heartier winter version.

1 cup vegetable broth (low-fat, low-sodium)
2 cans (540 mL) white kidney beans,
drained and rinsed
1/4 tsp dried thyme
1/4 tsp black pepper
2 cups baby spinach leaves, shredded
Pinch of salt

1. Bring the vegetable broth to a boil in a saucepan. Add the beans, thyme and black pepper. Simmer for about 10 minutes

2. Mash the bean mixture with a potato masher until fairly smooth. Stir in the spinach and salt until combined.

Makes 4 servings.

Vegetarian Moussaka

Traditionally made with ground lamb, moussaka can be made low-GI by using vegetables.

2 large eggplants (about 3 lbs total)
2 tsp salt
1 tsp canola oil
2 large onions, finely chopped
3 cloves garlic, minced
1 each red and green bell pepper, diced
1 tbsp dried oregano
1 tsp ground cinnamon
1/2 tsp black pepper
1/4 tsp ground allspice
1 can (796 mL) diced tomatoes
1/4 cup tomato paste
1 can (540 mL) chickpeas, drained and rinsed
1/4 cup chopped fresh flat-leaf parsley

Cheese Sauce:
2 tbsp canola oil
1/4 cup whole wheat flour
2 cups warm skim milk
1/4 tsp salt
Pinch each of nutmeg and black pepper
2/3 cup liquid egg
1/2 cup 1% pressed cottage cheese
1 cup crumbled light feta cheese

1. Preheat the oven to 425°F. Cut the eggplants into 4-inch-thick slices and layer them in a colander, sprinkling each layer with some of the salt. Let stand for 30 minutes, then rinse the slices and drain them well. Place them on baking sheets lined with parchment paper and roast, in batches if necessary, for about 20 minutes or until tender. Set aside.

2. Heat the oil in a large, shallow Dutch oven or deep nonstick skillet over medium heat. Add the onions, garlic, red and green peppers, oregano, cinnamon, pepper and allspice and cook until the onions have softened, about 5 minutes. Add the tomatoes and tomato paste and bring to a boil. Add the chickpeas and parsley, reduce the heat, and simmer for 15 minutes.

3. Make the Cheese Sauce: Heat the oil in a saucepan over medium heat. Stir in the flour and cook for 1 minute. Whisk in the milk and cook, whisking gently, for about 10 minutes or until the mixture is thick enough to coat the back of a spoon. Stir in the salt, nutmeg and black pepper. Let cool slightly and whisk in the egg and cottage cheese.

4. Preheat the oven to 350°F. Spread one-third of the tomato sauce on the bottom of a 9- × 13-inch baking dish. Top with one-third of the eggplant slices and one quarter of the feta cheese. Repeat the layers. After the last layer of eggplant, spread the cheese sauce evenly over the top and sprinkle with the remaining feta.

5. Bake for about 1 hour or until the top is golden brown. Let stand for 10 minutes before serving.

Makes 8 servings.

Roasted Vegetable Macaroni and Cheese

Macaroni and cheese is a favourite comfort food, so why not add some vegetables for flavour, colour and fibre?

2 carrots, coarsely chopped
2 zucchini, chopped
2 cloves garlic
1 small eggplant, cubed
1 red bell pepper, chopped
1 onion, cut into 8 wedges
1/4 cup vegetable broth (low-fat, low-sodium)
1 tsp dried thyme
1/2 tsp salt
1/4 tsp black pepper

Cheese Sauce:
3 tbsp canola oil
1/3 cup whole wheat flour
3 cups warm skim milk
2 tsp Dijon mustard
1 cup shredded light-style cheddar cheese
2 tbsp grated Parmesan cheese

1/4 tsp each salt and black pepper
1 1/2 cups whole wheat macaroni

1. Preheat the oven to 425°F. Toss together in a large bowl the carrots, zucchini, garlic, eggplant, red pepper, onion, vegetable broth, thyme, salt and pepper. Spread the mixture in a single layer on a large baking sheet lined with parchment paper or foil. Roast for about 35 minutes or until golden brown and tender-crisp. Set aside.

2. Bring a large pot of salted water to a boil.

3. Make the Cheese Sauce: Heat the oil in a large saucepan over medium-high heat. Add the flour and cook, stirring, for about 1 minute. Slowly whisk in the milk and continue whisking gently until the mixture is thick enough to coat the back of a spoon, about 5 minutes. Add the mustard, cheddar and Parmesan cheeses, salt and pepper and whisk until smooth. Remove from the heat.

4. Meanwhile, cook the macaroni in the boiling water until *al dente*, about 8 minutes. Drain well and add to the cheese sauce. Add the roasted vegetables and stir to combine.

Makes 4 to 6 servings.

Make Ahead: If you want to make this a day ahead, simply wrap the casserole dish before baking with plastic wrap and refrigerate. Remove the plastic wrap and bake in a 350°F oven for about 45 minutes or until heated through.

Roasted Pepper and Tomato Strata

Stratas are casseroles layered with bread. We've made ours green-light by using whole wheat bread and cutting back on the amount. This is a perfect make-ahead brunch or potluck dish.

8 slices whole wheat bread
2 jars (300 mL each) roasted red peppers, drained
4 cups chopped cooked broccoli
1 cup shredded light-style Swiss cheese
2 cups skim milk

1 cup liquid egg
2 tbsp Dijon mustard
2 tbsp chopped fresh flat-leaf parsley
1/4 tsp salt
1/4 tsp black pepper
2 tomatoes, sliced

1. Trim the crusts off the bread. Cut the slices into 6-inch cubes and sprinkle half over the bottom of a greased 9 × 13-inch baking dish.

2. Slice the peppers into long, thin strips. Sprinkle half of the peppers and half of the broccoli over the bread. Sprinkle with half of the cheese. Top with the remaining bread cubes, peppers, broccoli and cheese.

3. Whisk together in a large bowl the milk, liquid egg, mustard, parsley, salt and pepper. Pour over the bread mixture, cover and refrigerate for at least 2 hours or up to 24 hours.

4. Preheat the oven to 350°F. Place the tomato slices on top of the casserole, overlapping slightly if necessary. Bake, uncovered, for about 45 minutes or until edges are golden and a knife inserted in the centre comes out clean.

Makes 8 to 10 servings.

FISH AND SEAFOOD

Shrimp and Crab Cakes

These little cakes are brunch showstoppers. You can use scallops instead of the shrimp, and baby spinach for the arugula. However you choose to make them, these will disappear before your eyes.

1 can (540 mL) chickpeas, drained and rinsed
1 lb large raw shrimp, peeled and deveined
2 cups crabmeat
3/4 cup fresh whole wheat bread crumbs
1/3 cup liquid egg
1/2 cup finely chopped celery
1/4 cup chopped fresh dill
1/4 tsp salt
1/4 tsp black pepper
2 tomatoes, diced
2 red bell peppers, diced
3 tbsp chopped fresh flat-leaf parsley

Dressing:
1 tbsp extra-virgin olive oil
1 large clove garlic, peeled and minced
1/2 jalapeño pepper, minced
3 tbsp fresh lemon juice
4 cups torn arugula or spinach leaves

1. Place the chickpeas in a food processor and pulse until finely chopped. Scrape into a large bowl. Place the shrimp in the food processor and pulse until finely chopped. Add to the chickpeas.

2. Preheat the oven to 425°F. Place the crabmeat in a fine-mesh sieve and press out any liquid. Remove any cartilage if necessary and add the crabmeat to the bowl. Add the bread crumbs, liquid egg, celery, dill, salt and pepper, and use your hands to combine until the mixture sticks together. Form the batter into 18 cakes, each about 5-inch thick. Place the cakes on a baking sheet lined with parchment paper. Bake for about 20 minutes or until golden and firm to the touch.

3. Meanwhile, combine the tomatoes, red peppers and parsley in a bowl. Set aside.

4. Make the Dressing: Whisk together in a small bowl the oil, garlic, jalapeño and lemon juice. Set aside.

5. Arrange the arugula on a large serving platter and top with the shrimp and crab cakes. Sprinkle with the tomato mixture and drizzle the dressing over the top just before serving.

Makes 8 to 10 servings.

Quick Fish Steak with Tomato Chickpea Relish

This recipe is so versatile, you can use fish, chicken or turkey. The slight sweetness of the relish complements the peppery bite of the fish. It's perfect served with basmati rice and green beans.

Tomato Chickpea Relish:
2 large tomatoes, seeded and finely chopped
1 cup chopped cooked chickpeas
1/3 cup finely chopped red bell pepper
1/4 cup finely chopped onion
1/4 cup chopped fresh flat-leaf parsley
1/4 cup apple cider vinegar
1 tbsp sugar substitute
2 tsp pickling spice
Pinch each of salt and black pepper

Fish Steak:
1/4 cup red wine vinegar
2 tbsp chopped fresh thyme, or 1 tsp dried
2 cloves garlic, minced
2 tsp Dijon mustard
1/2 tsp black pepper
1 tuna steak (1 lb)

1. Preheat an outdoor grill or grill pan.

2. Make the Tomato Chickpea Relish: Stir together in a large bowl the tomatoes, chickpeas, red pepper, onion, parsley, vinegar, sugar substitute, pickling spice, salt and pepper. Set aside.

3. Stir together in a large, shallow dish the vinegar, thyme, garlic, mustard and pepper. Add the fish steak and turn to coat. Let marinate for 5 minutes.

4. Place the fish steak on the greased grill over medium-high heat and grill for about 8 minutes, turning once, or until medium rare (or cook to desired doneness).

5. Cut the fish steak into 4 pieces and serve with the relish.

Makes 4 servings.

Yellow-Light Lamb Option: Use 8 lean lamb chops in place of the fish steak. Increase the cooking time to 10 minutes for medium rare.

Green-Light Chicken Option: Use 4 chicken breasts, skinned, instead of the fish. Increase the cooking time to about 25 minutes.

Pan-Seared White Fish with Mandarin Salsa

A quick, bright citrusy salsa lends a tropical note to this hearty fish fillet. You can use tilapia, haddock or catfish for this elegant meal.

Mandarin Salsa:
2 cans (284 mL each) no-sugar-added mandarin oranges, drained
1 red bell pepper, diced
1/2 cup diced cucumber
1/4 cup finely diced red onion
3 tbsp chopped fresh cilantro
1 tbsp rice vinegar
1/4 tsp salt
Pinch of black pepper

Fish Fillets:
1/4 cup whole wheat flour
1/3 cup liquid egg
3/4 cup fresh whole wheat bread crumbs

1/4 cup chopped fresh flat-leaf parsley
2 tbsp wheat bran
2 tbsp wheat germ
1 tbsp chopped fresh tarragon, or 1 tsp dried
1/4 tsp salt
1/4 tsp black pepper
4 white fish fillets (4 oz each)
4 tsp canola oil

1. **Make the Mandarin Salsa:** Coarsely chop the mandarin slices and place them in a bowl. Add the red pepper, cucumber, onion, cilantro, rice vinegar, salt and pepper. Toss to combine.

2. **Prepare the Fish Fillets:** Prepare three large, shallow dishes. In the first, place the flour. In the second, place the liquid egg. In the third, combine the bread crumbs, parsley, wheat bran and germ, tarragon, salt and pepper. Dip a fish fillet into the flour first, shaking off the excess. Next, coat the fillet with liquid egg. Then dredge it evenly in the bread-crumb mixture. Repeat with the rest of the fillets. Place the prepared fillets on a plate lined with waxed paper and set aside.

3. Heat half of the oil in a large nonstick skillet over medium-high heat. Add 2 of the fillets and cook, turning once, or until golden brown, about 10 minutes. Repeat with the remaining oil and fillets. Serve topped with Mandarin Salsa.

Makes 4 servings.

POULTRY

Here are three easy-to-prepare chicken recipes that will become family favourites:

Asian Stir-Fry

2 servings
Vegetable oil cooking spray (preferably canola or olive oil)
3 cups chopped mixed vegetables, such as carrots, cauliflower, broccoli, mushrooms and snow peas (see Note below)
1 tsp grated fresh ginger
1 tsp soy sauce
Salt and black pepper
8 oz cooked skinless, boneless chicken breast or turkey breast

1. Spray oil in a nonstick skillet, then place it over medium heat.

2. Add the mixed vegetables and sauté until tender, about 5 minutes.

3. Add the ginger and soy sauce and stir to mix. Season to taste with salt and pepper.

4. Add the cooked chicken or turkey and stir to mix. Cook until the chicken or turkey is heated through, 2 minutes, then serve.

Variation: To prepare the stir-fry even more quickly, use 2 to 3 teaspoons of a light, store-bought stir-fry sauce in place of the fresh ginger, soy sauce, and salt and pepper.

Note: For convenience, use frozen mixed vegetables or frozen cut peppers.

Italian Chicken

2 servings
8 oz sliced mushrooms
1 medium onion, sliced
1 can (540 mL) chopped Italian tomatoes
1 clove garlic, minced
Chopped fresh or dried oregano and basil
8 oz cooked skinless, boneless chicken breast or turkey breast

1. Place the mushrooms, onion and tomatoes in a saucepan. Stir in a little water to prevent the tomatoes from sticking, and cook over medium-low heat until the mushrooms and onion are softened.

2. Add the garlic, oregano and basil, stir to mix, then simmer for 5 minutes.

3. Add the cooked chicken or turkey and stir to mix. Simmer until the chicken or turkey is heated through, 2 minutes, then serve.

Chicken Curry

2 servings
Vegetable oil cooking spray (preferably canola or olive oil)
1 medium onion, sliced
1 to 2 tsp curry powder, or to taste
1 cup sliced carrots
1 cup chopped celery
1/2 cup uncooked basmati rice
1 medium apple, chopped
1/4 cup raisins
8 oz cooked skinless, boneless chicken breast or turkey breast

1. Spray oil in a nonstick skillet, then place it over medium heat.

2. Add the onion and curry powder, stir to coat the onion with the curry, then sauté for 1 minute.

3. Add the carrots and celery, stir to mix, then sauté for 1 minute.

4. Add the rice, apple, raisins and 1 cup of water and stir to mix. Cover the skillet and let the curry simmer until all of the liquid is absorbed.

5. Add the cooked chicken or turkey and stir to mix. Cook until the chicken or turkey is heated through, 2 minutes, then serve.

Open-Faced Chicken Reuben Sandwich

The hefty Reuben sandwich has always been a big favourite with the lunch crowd at restaurants. This version is lightened up, packed with fibre and spiked with tangy spread. It's great for lunch or dinner served alongside a green salad.

Sandwich Spread:
1/2 cup plain yogurt
2 tsp balsamic vinegar
1 hard-boiled egg, finely chopped
2 tsp minced pitted green olives
2 tsp minced red bell pepper
1/2 tsp Worcestershire sauce
4 slices whole wheat bread
3 cups shredded cooked chicken (see Helpful Hint)
2 cups shredded cabbage
1 tomato, sliced
4 slices light-style Swiss cheese
2 tsp non-hydrogenated soft margarine or canola oil

1. Make the Sandwich Spread: Whisk together in a small bowl the yogurt, vinegar, egg, olives, red pepper and Worcestershire sauce.

2. Divide the spread between the 4 slices of bread. Top with chicken, cabbage and tomato. Place one slice of cheese on each sandwich.

3. Preheat the oven to 400°F.

4. Melt the margarine in a large ovenproof nonstick skillet over medium-high heat. Place the sandwiches in the skillet, in batches if necessary, and cook until the bread is toasted, about 5 minutes. Place the skillet in the oven until the cheese melts, about 5 minutes.

Makes 4 servings.

Helpful Hint: You can use leftover grilled or roasted chicken or turkey, or you can pick up 2 cooked chicken breasts at the grocery store; remove skin and any bones before using.

Basmati Rice Paella

This dish is a crowd pleaser—perfect for entertaining. Have a themed party with other Spanish foods such as wilted greens or stewed chickpeas.

1 tbsp extra-virgin olive oil
1 lb boneless, skinless chicken thighs
1 onion, chopped
4 cloves garlic, minced
1 red bell pepper, chopped
1 green bell pepper, chopped
4 cups chicken broth (low-fat, low-sodium)
1 can (796 mL) diced tomatoes
1 tbsp paprika
1/4 tsp saffron threads
1 1/2 cups basmati rice
8 oz green beans, trimmed
1 cup fresh or frozen lima beans
1 cup fresh or frozen peas
1 lb large raw shrimp, peeled and deveined
1 lb mussels, rinsed

1. Heat the oil in a large, shallow Dutch oven or a deep nonstick skillet over medium-high heat. Add the chicken pieces and cook on both sides until browned. Remove them to a plate.

2. Reduce the heat to medium. Add the onion, garlic and peppers and cook until the onion has softened, about 5 minutes. Add the chicken broth, tomatoes, paprika and saffron and bring to a boil. Stir in the rice, chicken and pan juices, reduce the heat to low, and simmer uncovered, gently, for about 20 minutes.

3. Meanwhile, cut the green beans into 1-inch pieces. Gently stir the beans, lima beans and peas into the rice mixture. Stir in the shrimp and mussels, cover, and cook for about 15 minutes or until the rice is tender and the mussels are open.

Makes 6 to 8 servings.

Helpful Hint: Before cooking, tap mussels gently on the counter to see if they will stay closed. Discard any mussels that don't stay closed. Also discard cooked mussels that remain closed after cooking.

Spinach-Stuffed Turkey Breast

Veggies are great on the side, but they also add tons of flavour and nutrition when served right in your meat. Try Swiss chard instead of the spinach in this recipe for a slightly sharper flavour.

1 tsp canola oil
1/2 cup chopped green onions
1 clove garlic, minced
1/2 red bell pepper, finely diced
1/2 yellow bell pepper, finely diced
1 cup cooked red kidney beans, mashed
1 tbsp finely chopped fresh ginger
2 cups chopped spinach
2 tbsp chopped fresh mint
1/4 tsp salt
1/4 tsp black pepper
1 boneless turkey breast (about 2 lbs)

Sesame Garlic Marinade:
3 tbsp soy sauce
2 tbsp rice vinegar
2 cloves garlic, minced
2 tsp sesame oil
1/2 tsp Asian chili paste or Tabasco sauce

1. Heat the oil in a large nonstick skillet over medium heat. Add the green onions and garlic and cook until the green onions begin to soften, about 3 minutes. Add the red and yellow peppers, beans and ginger, and cook, stirring, for 2 minutes. Add the spinach, cover, and cook, stirring occasionally, until wilted, about 5 minutes. Remove the skillet from the heat. Add the mint, salt and pepper. Let cool completely.

2. Remove the skin from the turkey and discard. Using a chef's knife, slice the turkey breast horizontally in half almost all the way through. Open the meat like a book and, using a meat mallet, pound the turkey to about 5-inch thick. Spread the spinach mixture over the turkey breast. Roll up the meat like a jelly roll, and, using kitchen string, tie the roll at 2-inch intervals. Place the tied roll in a small, shallow roasting pan.

3. Make the Sesame Garlic Marinade: Whisk together in a small bowl the soy sauce, rice vinegar, garlic, sesame oil and Asian chili paste. Pour the marinade over the turkey breast, turning to coat all sides. Cover with plastic wrap and refrigerate for at least 1 hour or for up to 4 hours.

4. Preheat the oven to 325°F. Roast the turkey for about 1 hour and 15 minutes or until a meat thermometer reaches 180°F. Let stand for 10 minutes before slicing into 5-inch-thick slices. Alternately, you can let the turkey cool completely, then refrigerate until cold. Cut into thin slices and serve.

Makes 6 to 8 servings.

Chicken Jambalaya

Jambalaya is a traditional Cajun dish in which rice is used to sop up the rich juices of the stew.

2 tsp canola oil
2 stalks celery, chopped
2 cloves garlic, minced
1 onion, chopped
1 lb boneless, skinless chicken, cut into 1/2-inch cubes
2 tsp dried thyme
2 tsp dried oregano
1 tsp chili powder
1/4 tsp cayenne pepper (optional)
2 cups chicken broth (low-fat, low-sodium)
2 green bell peppers, diced

1 can (796 mL) stewed tomatoes
1 can (540 mL) kidney beans, drained and rinsed
3/4 cup brown rice
1 bay leaf
1/4 cup chopped fresh flat-leaf parsley

1. Heat the oil in a Dutch oven over medium-high heat. Add the celery, garlic and onion and cook until the onion has softened, about 5 minutes. Add the chicken, thyme, oregano, chili powder and cayenne and cook, stirring, for 5 minutes.

2. Add the chicken broth, green peppers, tomatoes, kidney beans, rice, and bay leaf and bring to a boil. Reduce the heat to low, cover and simmer, stirring occasionally, for about 35 minutes or until the rice is tender. Let the dish stand for 5 minutes. Remove the bay leaf and discard. Stir in the parsley before serving.

Makes 4 servings.

Turkey Option: Use boneless, skinless turkey instead of the chicken.

Seafood Option: Add 8 oz of small raw shrimp, peeled and deveined, during the last 10 minutes of cooking.

MEAT

Chili and meat loaf are two traditional family pleasers, especially during the long winter months.

Chili

2 tsp olive oil
1 large onion, sliced
2 cloves of garlic, minced
1/2 lb extra-lean ground beef (optional)
2 green bell peppers, chopped
2 cups canned tomatoes
Chili powder to taste
1/2 tsp cayenne pepper (optional)
1/2 tsp salt
1/4 tsp basil
2 cups water
1 can (540 mL) red kidney beans, drained and rinsed
1 can (540 mL) white kidney beans, drained and rinsed
Chopped tomato, chopped fresh parsley and cilantro, and/or
  yogurt cheese (see below) for garnish (optional)

1. Warm the olive oil in a deep skillet or saucepan over medium heat. Add the onion and garlic and sauté until nearly tender.

2. Add the ground beef, if using, and cook until browned, breaking up the chunks with a spoon. Drain off any fat.

3. Add the bell peppers, tomatoes, chili powder, cayenne, if using, salt, basil and water and bring to a boil. Lower the heat and let simmer, uncovered, until the chili has reached the desired consistency, about 45 minutes.

4. Add the red and white kidney beans and cook over medium-low heat until heated through, about 5 minutes. Garnish the chili with tomato, parsley, cilantro and/or yogurt cheese if desired.

Makes 4 servings

Yogurt Cheese

Looking for a green-light alternative to sour cream? Try yogurt cheese—it's easy to make your own from plain nonfat yogurt. Place a sieve lined with cheesecloth, paper towels or a coffee filter over a bowl. Spoon the yogurt into the sieve and cover it with plastic wrap. Place the sieve and bowl in the refrigerator. Let the yogurt drain overnight—the next day you will have yogurt cheese.

Meat Loaf

1 1/2 lbs extra-lean ground beef (less than 10 percent fat)
1 cup tomato juice
1/2 cup old-fashioned rolled oats (uncooked)
1 egg, lightly beaten
1/2 cup chopped onion
1 tbsp Worcestershire sauce
1/2 tsp salt (optional)
1/4 tsp black pepper

1. Preheat the oven to 350°F.

2. In a large bowl, combine all ingredients. Mix lightly but thoroughly.

3. Press the meat loaf mixture into an 8 × 4-inch loaf pan.

4. Bake the meat loaf for 1 hour, or until an instant-read meat thermometer inserted into the centre registers 160°F.

5. Let the meat loaf stand for 5 minutes before draining off any juices and slicing it.

Makes 6 servings

Variation: Extra-lean ground beef is still relatively high in fat. A lower-fat and better alternative to ground beef is an equal amount of ground turkey or chicken breast. When fully cooked, ground turkey or chicken will register 170°F on an instant-read meat thermometer.

Spaghetti and Meatballs

A home-cooked meal is a wonderful thing to come home to, and this one is a favourite of many. You can make the meatballs ahead and freeze them.

1 egg
1/3 cup fresh whole wheat bread crumbs
1/4 cup wheat bran
1/4 cup chopped fresh flat-leaf parsley
1 clove garlic, minced
1/4 tsp salt
1/4 tsp black pepper
12 oz lean ground turkey or chicken
2 cups low-fat chunky vegetable pasta sauce
1 cup cooked chickpeas
1/2 green bell pepper, diced
6 oz whole wheat spaghetti

1. Preheat the oven to 350°F.

2. In a large bowl, stir together the egg, bread crumbs, bran, parsley, garlic, salt and pepper. Using your hands, gently work in the ground turkey until well combined. Roll the mixture into 1-inch round meatballs and place on a baking sheet lined with aluminum foil. Bake for about 12 minutes or until no longer pink inside.

3. Meanwhile, bring a large pot of salted water to a boil.

4. In a separate large saucepan, cook the pasta sauce, chickpeas and green pepper over medium heat. Add the meatballs and simmer for 15 minutes.

5. Cook the pasta in the boiling water until *al dente*, about 10 minutes. Remove the meatballs to a small serving bowl. Drain the pasta and add it to the pasta sauce, tossing to coat well. Serve with the meatballs.

Makes 4 servings.

Make Ahead: Cool meatballs completely and freeze in an airtight container for up to 2 months.

Helpful Hint: To make your own pasta sauce, purée 2 cans (796 mL each) plum tomatoes. Place in a saucepan over medium heat along with 1 onion, chopped; 2 cloves garlic, minced; 1 zucchini, chopped; 1 red bell pepper, chopped; 2 tsp dried oregano; and 1 tsp each salt and black pepper. Bring to a boil and simmer for about 40 minutes or until thickened slightly. Keep refrigerated for up to 1 week or freeze for up to 1 month.

Baked Beans

Normally, baked beans are packed with sugar and molasses, which add lots of calories. Our version achieves the same comforting, filling and fibre-packed dish without the sugar.

2 cups dry navy or small white beans
8 cups water
1 can (796 mL) diced tomatoes
4 oz lean Black Forest ham, chopped
1 large red onion, finely chopped
1 can (156 mL) tomato paste
1/4 cup brown sugar substitute
2 tbsp Dijon mustard
1 tbsp Worcestershire sauce
2 tsp Tabasco sauce
1/2 tsp salt
1/2 tsp black pepper

1. Rinse the beans and place them in a Dutch oven filled with water. Cover, and let soak overnight. The next day, drain and rinse the beans.

2. In the same pot, add the 8 cups of water and the beans and bring to a boil. Reduce the heat, cover, and simmer, stirring occasionally, for about 1 1/2 hours or until the beans are tender. Drain the beans, reserving the cooking liquid.

3. Preheat the oven to 300°F.

4. In the same Dutch oven, combine 1 cup of the reserved cooking liquid, the beans, tomatoes, ham, onion, tomato paste, brown sugar substitute, mustard, Worcestershire sauce, Tabasco, salt and pepper. Cover and bake, stirring occasionally, for 2 1/2 hours. Uncover, and cook for 1 hour or until thickened.

Makes 8 servings.

Quick-Soak Option: Rinse the beans and place them in a Dutch oven filled with water. Bring to a boil and cook for 2 minutes. Cover, remove from the heat, and let sit for an hour. Then drain and continue with the recipe.

Slow-Cooker Option: Place the cooked beans with the rest of the ingredients in a slow cooker and cook on Low for 8 to 10 hours or on High for 4 to 6 hours or until tender.

Sloppy Joes

Here's a meal that is great for lunch or dinner after a weekend hockey game or on a cold winter night. Serve it with cut veggies and hummus for dipping.

1 lb extra-lean ground beef
1 onion, chopped
4 cloves garlic, minced
1 green bell pepper, chopped
1/2 jalapeño pepper, minced
1 can (540 mL) red kidney beans, drained and rinsed
1 can (796 mL) diced tomatoes
1/4 cup old-fashioned rolled oats
1 tbsp chili powder
2 tsp Worcestershire sauce
4 whole wheat pita halves
2 cups chopped romaine or iceberg lettuce
2 tomatoes, chopped

1. Cook the beef in a large, deep nonstick skillet or Dutch oven over medium-high heat until browned, about 8 minutes. Add the onion, garlic, green pepper, and jalapeño pepper and cook for 5 minutes. Add the beans, tomatoes, oats, chili powder and Worcestershire sauce and bring to a boil. Reduce the heat and simmer, stirring occasionally, until thickened, about 25 minutes.

2. Scoop the sloppy joe mixture into pita halves and top with lettuce and tomato.

Makes 4 to 6 servings.

Lighter Option: You can use ground turkey or chicken instead of beef.

Vegetarian Option: You can use ground meat substitute instead of the beef.

Chili Option: To serve this as a chili, simply reduce the cooking time to about 15 minutes.

Steak Fettuccine

A steak with a serving of pasta sounds like old-fashioned, fattening fare. Not our version. The meat is marinated with a peppery dressing and served, sliced, atop fettuccine dressed with a fresh tomato sauce. The result is light and flavourful, yet elegant enough for company.

1 top sirloin grilling steak (1 lb)
2 tbsp Dijon mustard
2 tsp dried Italian herb seasoning
1/2 tsp black pepper
Salt
1 tsp extra-virgin olive oil
2 shallots, thinly sliced
2 cloves garlic, minced
1 tsp dried oregano
1/2 tsp dried basil
3 tomatoes, chopped
1 red bell pepper, thinly sliced
1 orange bell pepper, thinly sliced
1/2 cup beef broth (low-fat, low-sodium)
1 cup snow peas, trimmed
6 oz whole wheat fettuccine or linguine

1. Preheat an outdoor grill or grill pan. *Trim all fat from the steak and discard.*

2. In a small bowl, stir together the mustard, Italian herb seasoning and black pepper. Spread evenly over the steak. Place the steak on the greased grill over medium-high heat and grill for about 8 minutes, turning once, or until medium rare. Remove to a plate, cover, and keep warm.

3. Meanwhile, bring a large pot of salted water to a boil.

4. Heat the oil in a nonstick skillet over medium-high heat. Add the shallots, garlic, oregano and basil and cook until the shallots start to become golden, about 5 minutes. Add the tomatoes, bell peppers and broth, and bring to a boil. Reduce the heat and simmer gently until the tomatoes start to break down, about 5 minutes. Add the snow peas and cook until bright green, about 3 minutes. Stir in 1/4 tsp salt.

5. Cook the fettuccine in the boiling salted water until *al dente*, about 10 minutes. Drain well and return the pasta to the pot. Toss with the sauce to coat. Place the pasta in a large serving dish. Thinly slice the steak across the grain and lay on top of the fettuccine. Serve immediately.

Makes 4 servings.

Classic Meat Lasagna

In a traditional lasagna, cheese adds a delicious creamy layer— as well as a lot of calories. You can get that same rich flavour with a green-light béchamel sauce.

1 lb extra-lean ground beef or veal
1 onion, finely chopped
4 cloves garlic, minced
8 oz mushrooms, sliced
2 zucchini, trimmed and chopped
1 each red and green bell pepper, chopped
1 tbsp dried oregano
1/2 tsp red pepper flakes
1/2 cup beef broth (low-fat, low-sodium)
2 cans (796 mL each) plum tomatoes, puréed
1/4 tsp each salt and black pepper
12 whole wheat lasagna noodles

Béchamel Sauce:
1/4 cup canola oil
1/2 cup whole wheat flour
4 cups warm skim milk
2 tbsp grated Parmesan cheese
1/4 tsp each salt and black pepper
Pinch of nutmeg

1. Cook the ground beef, onion and garlic in a deep nonstick skillet over medium heat until browned, about 8 minutes. Add the mushrooms, zucchini, bell peppers, oregano and red pepper flakes, and cook, stirring occasionally, until the onion has softened, about 10 minutes. Add the broth and bring to a boil. Cook until all the liquid has evaporated, then add the puréed tomatoes, salt and pepper, and bring to a boil again. Reduce the heat and simmer until thickened, about 30 minutes.

2. Bring a large pot of salted water to a boil.

3. **Make the Béchamel Sauce:** Heat the oil in a saucepan over medium-high heat. Add the flour and cook, stirring, for 1 minute. Slowly pour in the milk and whisk to combine. Cook, whisking gently, until the mixture thickens, about 5 minutes. Add the Parmesan cheese, salt, pepper and nutmeg. Remove from the heat.

4. Meanwhile, cook the lasagna noodles in the boiling water until *al dente*, about 10 minutes. Drain, and rinse under cold water. Lay the noodles flat on damp tea towels and set aside.

5. Preheat the oven to 350°F.

6. Ladle 1 1/2 cups of the meat sauce in the bottom of a 9 × 13-inch glass baking dish. Lay 3 noodles on top of the sauce. Spread with another 1 cup of the meat sauce, then one-quarter of the béchamel sauce. Repeat the layers—noodles, meat sauce, béchamel sauce—ending with béchamel sauce. Cover the dish with aluminum foil and place it on a baking sheet. Bake for 45 minutes, then uncover and bake for 15 minutes or until bubbly. Cool 10 minutes before serving.

Makes 8 servings.

SNACKS

Over-the-Top Bran Muffins with Pear

These muffins are big and full of fibre. They are "Over-the-Top" because they rise above the top of the pan, so be sure to grease the top of your muffin pan too. The addition of fresh, chopped pear keeps these muffins moist.

1 cup All-Bran or 100% Bran cereal
1 cup wheat bran
1 1/2 cups plain low-fat yogurt
2 cups whole wheat flour
1/2 cup brown sugar substitute
1 tbsp baking powder
2 tsp baking soda
1/4 tsp salt
1/2 cup skim milk
1/4 cup canola oil
1 egg
2 tsp vanilla extract
2 pears, cored and diced

1. Preheat the oven to 375°F.

2. Combine the cereal and wheat bran in a bowl. Stir in the yogurt and let stand for 10 minutes.

3. In a separate bowl, combine the flour, brown sugar substitute, baking powder, baking soda and salt.

4. Add the milk, oil, egg and vanilla to the bran mixture and stir to combine. Pour over the flour mixture and stir until just combined. Stir in the pear.

5. Divide the batter between 12 greased or paper-lined muffin cups. Bake until the tops are golden and firm to the touch, about 25 minutes. Let cool on a rack for 5 minutes. Remove the muffins from the pan and let cool completely.

Makes 12 muffins.

Dried Fruit Option: Use 1 cup dried cranberries, raisins, diced apricots or dried blueberries instead of the pear.

Blueberry Option: Use 2 cups fresh blueberries instead of the pear.

Storage: Wrap each muffin individually in plastic wrap and freeze in an airtight container for up to 1 month or keep at room temperature in an airtight container for up to 3 days.

Apple Bran Muffins

My wife, Ruth, created this recipe several years ago when I was trying to lose weight. We'd make large batches of them and freeze them. Then, whenever I needed a snack, I'd warm one in the microwave. They are so convenient and delicious.

Vegetable oil cooking spray
3/4 cup All-Bran or Bran Buds cereal
1 cup skim milk
2/3 cup whole wheat flour
1/3 cup sugar substitute
2 tsp baking powder
1/2 tsp baking soda
1/4 tsp salt
1 tsp ground allspice
1/2 tsp ground cloves
1 1/2 cups oat bran
2/3 cup raisins
1 large apple, peeled and cut into 1/4-inch cubes
1 omega-3 egg, lightly beaten
2 tsp vegetable oil
1/2 cup applesauce (unsweetened)

1. Preheat the oven to 350°F. Spray a 12-cup muffin tin with vegetable oil cooking spray.

2. Mix the cereal and skim milk in a bowl and let stand for a few minutes.

3. In a large bowl, mix the flour, sugar substitute, baking powder, baking soda, salt, allspice and cloves. Stir in the oat bran, raisins and apple.

4. In a small bowl, combine the egg, oil and applesauce. Stir egg mixture and bran mixture into the dry ingredients.

5. Spoon the batter into the prepared muffin tin. Bake until lightly browned, about 20 minutes.

Makes 12 muffins.

Homemade Granola Bars

These bars are very nutritious and really satisfying.

1 1/3 cups whole wheat flour
1/3 cup sugar substitute
2 tsp baking powder
1/4 cup All-Bran or Bran Buds cereal
1 tsp each ground cinnamon and allspice
1/2 tsp each ground ginger and salt
1 1/2 cups old-fashioned rolled oats
1 cup finely chopped dried apricots
1/2 cup shelled sunflower seeds
3/4 cup applesauce (unsweetened)
1/2 cup apple juice (unsweetened)
3 omega-3 eggs
2 tsp vegetable oil

1. Preheat the oven to 400°F. Line a shallow 8 × 12-inch baking dish with parchment paper.

2. Mix the flour, sugar substitute, baking powder, cereal, cinnamon, allspice, ginger and salt in a large bowl. Stir in the oats, apricots and sunflower seeds.

3. Mix the applesauce, apple juice, eggs and oil, and add to the flour mixture. Pour the batter into the prepared baking dish and spread it out evenly.

4. Bake until lightly browned, 15 to 20 minutes. Let cool and cut into 16 bars.

Makes 16 bars.

Oatcakes

These Scottish treats have been around for a long time. Traditionally they were made without sweetening, but over time the sweetened version appeared and people were hooked. You can try these without the sugar substitute and see which version you prefer.

2 cups old-fashioned rolled oats
1 cup whole wheat flour
1/2 cup wheat bran
1/3 cup sugar substitute
1/2 tsp salt
1/2 cup non-hydrogenated soft margarine
1 egg, lightly beaten
3 tbsp water

1. Combine the oats, flour, bran, sugar substitute and salt in a large bowl. Use a wooden spoon to stir in the margarine until a crumbly mixture forms. Add the egg and water and stir until the dough sticks together.

2. Preheat the oven to 350°F. Divide the dough into 16 pieces. Form each piece into a 1/4-inch-thick round and place on a baking sheet lined with parchment paper. Bake for 15 minutes. Turn the oatcakes over and bake on the other side until firm and golden, about 10 minutes.

Makes 16 oatcakes.

Blueberry Bars

This breakfast bar spinoff contains much more fibre and far fewer calories than store-bought ones. You can make them on the weekend to snack on throughout the week.

2 1/2 cups frozen blueberries
1/4 cup water
2 tbsp sugar substitute
1/2 tsp grated lemon zest
2 tsp fresh lemon juice
1 tbsp cornstarch
1 cup old-fashioned rolled oats
3/4 cup whole wheat flour
3/4 cup wheat bran
1/2 cup brown sugar substitute
1/4 tsp baking soda
1/2 cup soft non-hydrogenated margarine
3 tbsp liquid egg

1. Bring the blueberries, water, sugar substitute, lemon zest and juice, and cornstarch to a boil in a saucepan over medium heat. Cook, stirring, until thickened and bubbly, about 2 minutes. Let cool.

2. Preheat the oven to 350°F.

3. Combine the oats, flour, bran, brown sugar substitute and baking soda in a bowl. Use a wooden spoon to work in the margarine until the mixture resembles coarse crumbs. Add the liquid egg and stir until moistened. Reserve 3/4 cup of the mixture for the top. Press the remaining mixture into the bottom of an 8-inch baking pan lined with parchment paper. Spread with blueberry filling. Sprinkle with the reserved oat mixture.

4. Bake until the crust is golden and the blueberry filling is bubbly at the edges, about 30 minutes. Let cool completely before cutting into bars.

Makes 24 bars.

Storage: Place bars in an airtight container and keep refrigerated for up to 5 days or freeze for up to 2 weeks.

DESSERTS

Oatmeal Cookies

These soft cookies make a homey afternoon snack with a glass of milk. They are also perfect for lunch bags. Kids and adults alike are always happy to find a cookie in their brown bags.

2 cups old-fashioned rolled oats
3/4 cup whole wheat flour
1/2 cup wheat bran
1/2 tsp baking soda
1/2 tsp ground cinnamon
Pinch of salt
1 cup brown sugar substitute
1/2 cup non-hydrogenated soft margarine
1/4 cup liquid egg
1/4 cup water
2 tsp vanilla extract
1/2 cup dried currants (optional)

1. Preheat the oven to 375°F.

2. In a large bowl, stir together the oats, flour, bran, baking soda, cinnamon and salt. Set aside.

3. In another large bowl, beat the brown sugar substitute, margarine, liquid egg, water and vanilla until smooth. Stir the oat mixture into the margarine mixture until combined. Add the currants, if using, and stir to combine.

4. Drop the dough by heaping tablespoonfuls onto a baking sheet lined with parchment paper and flatten slightly. Bake until firm and golden on bottom, about 8 minutes. Repeat with the remaining dough. Let cool on a rack.

Makes about 28 cookies.

Storage: Keep in an airtight container for up to 3 days or freeze for up to 1 month.

Chewy Peanut Bars

Here's a chewy granola treat that's sure to be a hit with the whole family.

1 1/2 cups old-fashioned rolled oats
1/4 cup chopped unsalted peanuts (optional)
1/2 cup wheat bran
1/3 cup whole wheat flour
1/2 tsp each baking soda and baking powder
Pinch each of salt and ground cinnamon
2/3 cup liquid egg
1/2 cup smooth peanut butter (natural, no sugar added)
1/4 cup brown sugar substitute
2 tsp vanilla extract

1. Preheat the oven to 350°F.

2. In a large bowl, combine the oats, peanuts (if using), wheat bran, flour, baking soda, baking powder, salt and cinnamon.

3. In another bowl, beat the liquid egg, peanut butter, brown sugar substitute and vanilla until combined. Add the oat mixture and stir to combine. Scrape the dough into an 8-inch square baking pan lined with parchment paper. With damp hands, press down the mixture to flatten evenly. Bake until firm to the touch, about 12 minutes. Let cool and cut into bars.

Makes 12 bars.

Chocolate Drop Cookies

These moist cookies are wonderful dunked into a glass of milk. Though beans might seem an odd addition, trust us, they keep the batter tender and sneak in some extra fibre.

1/2 cup cooked white kidney beans
1 tbsp wheat bran
1/4 cup plus 2 tbsp skim milk
1/3 cup non-hydrogenated soft margarine
3/4 cup whole wheat flour
1/2 cup sugar substitute

1/3 cup unsweetened cocoa powder
1 egg
2 tsp vanilla extract
1/2 tsp baking soda

1. Preheat the oven to 375°F.

2. Put the white kidney beans, wheat bran, and 2 tbsp skim milk into a food processor and purée until well blended. Set aside.

3. In a large bowl, beat the margarine, flour, sugar substitute, bean purée, cocoa powder, the remaining skim milk, egg, vanilla and baking soda until combined.

4. Drop the batter by tablespoons onto a baking sheet lined with parchment paper. Bake until firm to the touch, about 10 minutes. Let cool on a rack.

Makes about 24 cookies.

Chocolate Almond Slices

These are similar to biscotti in that they are baked twice. Adults and kids love them and they keep well. You can add 1/4 cup of dried cranberries or raisins for some colour and extra flavour, if desired.

1/4 cup non-hydrogenated soft margarine
1/2 cup sugar substitute
1/2 cup liquid egg
4 tsp vanilla extract
1/4 tsp almond extract (optional)
1/2 cup unsweetened cocoa
1/2 cup wheat bran
1/4 cup wheat germ
1/2 cup whole wheat flour
2 tsp baking powder
Pinch of salt
1/2 cup slivered almonds

1. Preheat the oven to 350°F.

2. In a large bowl, cream together the margarine and sugar substitute. Beat in the liquid egg, vanilla and almond extract, if using. Beat in the cocoa, wheat bran, wheat germ, half of the flour, baking powder and salt. Stir in the remaining flour and gently mix in the almonds with your hands.

3. Shape the dough into 2 logs, each about 10 inches long, and place them on a baking sheet lined with parchment paper. Flatten each slightly.

4. Bake for about 20 minutes or until firm. Let the pan cool on a rack for about 15 minutes.

5. Turn the oven down to 300°F. Use a knife to cut each log diagonally into 1/2-inch slices. Place the slices on a baking sheet, cut sides down. Bake, turning once, until crisp, about 15 minutes. Let cool completely before serving.

Makes about 2 dozen cookies.

Storage: Keep in a resealable plastic bag or airtight container at room temperature for up to 5 days or freeze for up to 1 month.

Fruit and Yogurt Parfaits

Enjoy these parfaits for breakfast, dessert or a snack. Use whatever fruit is seasonal—blueberries, strawberries and apples all work well.

2 cups old-fashioned rolled oats
1/2 cup wheat germ
1/3 cup wheat bran
1/4 cup slivered almonds
1/4 cup shelled unsalted sunflower seeds
2 tbsp sugar substitute
1 tbsp canola oil
1 tbsp water
2 tsp grated orange zest
1 tsp vanilla extract
Pinch of salt
1/2 cup raisins or dried cranberries

1 tub (750 g) nonfat, fruit-flavoured yogurt with sugar
  substitute
2 cups chopped fresh fruit or berries

1. Preheat the oven to 300°F.

2. In a large bowl, toss together the oats, wheat germ and bran, almonds and sunflower seeds.

3. In a small bowl, whisk together the sugar substitute, oil, water, orange zest, vanilla and salt. Pour over the oat mixture and toss well to coat evenly. Spread the mixture onto a large baking sheet lined with parchment paper and bake, stirring once, until golden brown, about 30 minutes. Let cool completely. Add the raisins, stirring to combine.

4. In a glass serving bowl, layer 1 cup of the yogurt then half of the granola. Repeat once and top with the remaining yogurt. Sprinkle the fruit on top.

Makes 6 servings.

Storage: Cover and refrigerate for up to 2 days. Note that as the parfait sits, the granola softens.

Granola Storage: Keep in a resealable plastic bag or airtight container at room temperature for up to 3 days.

Yogurt Cheese Option: Use yogurt cheese (page 131) instead of yogurt.

Crustless Fruit-Topped Cheesecake

The best part of cheesecake is the rich filling, so we've eliminated the crust and focused on the middle and top layers. You can change the topping according to which fruit is in season.

1 tub (500 g) 1% cottage cheese
1 package (250 g) light cream cheese, softened
1 cup nonfat, fruit-flavoured yogurt with sugar substitute
3/4 cup sugar substitute
1/4 cup cornstarch

2 egg whites
1 tbsp vanilla extract
Pinch of salt

Fruit Topping:
4 cups fresh raspberries, blueberries or sliced strawberries
2 tsp fresh lemon juice
Sugar substitute

1. Preheat the oven to 325°F.

2. Purée the cottage cheese in a food processor or blender until very smooth. Add the cream cheese and purée until the mixture is smooth. Add the yogurt, sugar substitute, cornstarch, egg whites, vanilla and salt and purée until smooth.

3. Pour the batter into a greased and parchment-lined 8- or 9-inch springform pan. Wrap the bottom and sides of the pan with aluminum foil. Place in a large roasting pan and fill the roasting pan with hot water to come halfway up the sides of the springform pan.

4. Bake until the centre is slightly jiggly when the pan is tapped, about 40 minutes. Turn the oven off and run a small knife around the edge of the pan. Let the cake stand in the cooling oven for about 30 minutes more. Remove to a rack and let cool to room temperature. Cover, and refrigerate until chilled, about 2 hours.

5. **Make Fruit Topping:** Meanwhile, in a large bowl combine the raspberries, lemon juice and sugar substitute to taste. Cut the cheesecake into wedges and pour the fruit topping over.

Makes 8 servings.

Storage: Keep the cheesecake covered and refrigerated for up to 3 days.

Almond-Crusted Pears

This dessert makes an elegant ending at a dinner party. The crunchy almond crust contrasts nicely with the tender flesh of the pears.

Yogurt Cheese:
1 cup plain low-fat yogurt
4 tbsp sugar substitute
1/2 tsp grated orange zest (optional)
3/4 cup sliced almonds
2 tbsp wheat germ
4 ripe Bartlett or Bosc pears, cored
2 tbsp liquid egg
1/2 cup pear nectar or juice

1. Make the Yogurt Cheese: Place the yogurt in a sieve lined with paper towels or a coffee filter. Place the sieve over a bowl. Cover with plastic wrap and refrigerate for at least 1 hour or for up to 4 hours. Discard the liquid that drains off and transfer the yogurt cheese to another bowl. Add 2 tbsp of the sugar substitute and the orange zest and stir to combine. Cover with plastic wrap and refrigerate.

2. Preheat the oven to 400°F.

3. Use your hands to crush the almonds slightly, then place them in a shallow dish. Add the wheat germ and the remaining sugar substitute and stir to combine.

4. Fill the pears loosely with the almond mixture. Brush each pear with a light coating of liquid egg, then roll and press the pears into the almond mixture. Place the coated pears in an 8-inch square baking dish, standing upright. Pour the pear nectar in the bottom of the dish and sprinkle any remaining almond mixture into the pan. Cover the dish lightly with aluminum foil and bake until a knife slips easily into the pears, about 30 minutes. Remove the foil and bake until the crust is golden and the juices have thickened, about 10 minutes. Let cool slightly. Serve the pears with some of the juice from the pan and the yogurt cheese.

Makes 4 servings.

Fruit-Filled Pavlova

Pavlovas are meringues filled with whipped cream and fruit.
We use tofu and yogurt cheese in place of the whipped
cream—delicious!

8 egg whites
1/2 tsp cream of tartar
Pinch of salt
3/4 cup sugar substitute
2 tbsp cornstarch
2 tsp vanilla extract

Fruit Filling:
1 package (300 g) soft silken tofu, drained
1 cup yogurt cheese (page 131)
1/4 cup sugar substitute
1/2 tsp grated orange zest
4 cups mixed fruit (such as fresh berries, orange sections and
  peach wedges)
2 tbsp chopped fresh mint

1. Preheat the oven to 275°F.

2. Put the egg whites in a large bowl and beat with an electric
mixer until frothy. Add the cream of tartar and salt and beat
until soft peaks form. Gradually add the sugar substitute and
beat until the peaks become stiff. Beat in the cornstarch and
vanilla to combine.

3. Spread the mixture into an 8-inch round on a baking sheet
lined with parchment paper. Mound the edges slightly higher
than the centre to form a shell. Bake until lightly golden, about
40 minutes. Turn off the oven and let the meringue rest in the
oven for 1 hour. Remove to a large serving platter.

4. Make the Fruit Filling: Meanwhile, combine in a large bowl
the tofu, yogurt cheese, sugar substitute and orange zest.
Scrape into the meringue shell and top with the fruit mixture.
Sprinkle with mint before serving.

Makes 8 to 10 servings.

*Storage: The pavlova shell can be made up to 4 hours ahead. Fill
it with the fruit filling no more than 1 hour before serving.*

Frozen Blueberry Treat

This tangy, refreshing yogurt treat tastes like blueberry sorbet. Use an ice cream machine if you have one.

1/2 cup water
1/2 cup sugar substitute
3 cups fresh blueberries
1 cup low-fat plain yogurt

1. In a saucepan over medium heat, bring the water and sugar substitute to a boil. Remove from the heat and let cool completely.

2. Meanwhile, purée the blueberries in a food processor or blender. Add the yogurt and pulse to combine. Add the sugar substitute–water mixture and pulse to combine. Pour into an 8- or 9-inch metal pan and freeze until firm, about 2 hours. Cut into chunks and, working quickly, place batches of the frozen chunks in the food processor. Purée until smooth, scrape into an airtight container and refreeze until firm.

3. Before serving, place the frozen treat in the refrigerator for 15 minutes to soften slightly.

Makes about 3 cups.

Storage: Keep tightly covered in the freezer for up to 1 week.

A SAMPLE ONE-WEEK GREEN-LIGHT MENU PLAN

Breakfast	Oatmeal (page 94)
	Tea or decaffeinated coffee
Snack	Apple Bran Muffin (page 139)
	Glass of skim milk
Lunch	Niçoise Salad (page 107)
	1 slice whole wheat bread
Snack	1% cottage cheese with orange sections and a few almonds
Dinner	Classic Meat Lasagna (pages 136–37)
	Green salad
	Frozen Blueberry Treat (page 151)
Snack	Homemade Granola Bar (page 140)
	Glass of skim milk

TUESDAY:

Breakfast	Homemade Muesli (pages 94–95)
	Orange
	Tea or decaffeinated coffee
Snack	1 Chocolate Almond Slice (pages 145–46)
	Pear slices
	Glass of skim milk
Lunch	Cauliflower and Chickpea Soup (page 102)
	1 slice whole wheat bread with 4 oz turkey breast, mustard, cucumber, tomato and lettuce
Snack	Laughing Cow Light cheese with celery, carrots and cherry tomatoes
Dinner	Chicken Jambalaya (pages 128–29)
	Basmati rice

Green salad

Berries and nonfat yogurt

Snack   2 Oatmeal Cookies (page 143)

Glass of skim milk

WEDNESDAY:

Breakfast   Homemade Muesli (pages 94–95)

Tea or decaffeinated coffee

Snack   Laughing Cow cheese with grapes

2 high fibre crackers

Glass of skim milk

Lunch   Waldorf Chicken and Rice Salad (page 105)

Grapes

Snack   Homemade Granola Bar (page 140)

Glass of skim milk

Dinner   Sloppy Joes (page 134)

Hummus with cucumber, broccoli and
    bell pepper slices

fruit and non-fat yogurt

Snack   1 Chocolate Almond Slice (pages 145–46)

Glass of skim milk

THURSDAY:

Breakfast   Oatmeal (page 94)

Tea or decaffeinated coffee

Snack   Over-the-Top Bran Muffin with Pear
    (page 138)

Glass of skim milk

Lunch   Shrimp Caesar Salad (pages 109–10)

Canned peaches in juice

Snack   Laughing Cow Light cheese with 2 Wasa
    Fibre Crispbreads

Dinner   Asian Stir-Fry (page 123)

Basmati rice

Fruit and Yogurt Parfait (page 146)

Snack   1 Blueberry Bar (page 142)

Glass of skim milk

FRIDAY:

Breakfast   Homemade Muesli (pages 94–95)

Orange

Tea or decaffeinated coffee

Snack   1 Chocolate Almond Slice (pages 145–146)

Apple slices

Glass of skim milk

Lunch   Mixed Bean Salad (page 104)

Grapes

Snack   1% cottage cheese with fruit and almonds

Dinner   Pan-Seared White Fish with Mandarin
          Salsa (pages 121–22)

Boiled new or small potatoes

Green beans

Green salad

1/2 cup low-fat, no-added-sugar ice cream

Snack   Over-the-Top Bran Muffin with Pear
          (page 138)

Glass of skim milk

SATURDAY:

Breakfast   Mexican Omelette (pages 95–96)

Grapefruit slices

Tea or decaffeinated coffee

Snack   Nonfat fruit yogurt sprinkled with Bran Buds

Lunch   Open-Faced Chicken Reuben Sandwich
          (pages 125–26)

Small green salad

	Glass of skim milk
Snack	1 Blueberry Bar (page 142)
	Glass of skim milk
Dinner	Steak Fettuccine (pages 135–36)
	Green salad
	Fruit-filled Pavlova (page 150)
Snack	2 Oatmeal Cookies (page 143)
	Glass of skim milk

SUNDAY:

Breakfast	Green Eggs and Ham (pages 99–100)
	Tea or decaffeinated coffee
Snack	Laughing Cow Light cheese with 2 Wasa Fibre Crispbreads
Lunch	Bean and Onion Pizza (pages 112–13)
	Small green salad
	Pear
	Glass of skim milk
Snack	Hummus with cucumber and baby carrots
Dinner	Spinach-Stuffed Turkey Breast (pages 127–28)
	Boiled new or small potatoes
	Broccoli
	Green salad
	Almond-Crusted Pears (page 149)
Snack	Homemade Granola Bar (page 140)
	Glass of skim milk

More delicious recipes can be found in *The G.I. Diet Cookbook.*

Chapter 10
Eating Out

One of the most difficult challenges when trying to lose weight is eating away from home. You lose much of the control over content and preparation that you enjoy at home. However, as you will see, with a little care you can still eat the green-light way.

Dining out is often a social occasion with family, friends or co-workers, and you don't want to be a party pooper by making everyone feel uncomfortable with your dietary concerns. There is the risk of fellow diners egging you on to "live a little," which usually means poor food choices, extra drinks and decadent desserts. The best solution is to be upfront that you are trying to improve your health by reducing your weight. Solicit their support.

FAST FOOD

Most of the leading fast-food restaurants have introduced menu items that are lower in fat and calories. Beware of the amount of sodium (salt) that is often added to offset any perceived flavour loss. Remember, salt retains liquid, which is the last thing you need when you're trying to lose weight and trying to keep your blood pressure in check. If you are not sure about salt levels in the food, ask your server for a nutritional information sheet, provided by most family and fast-food restaurant chains.

A COUPLE OF GROUND RULES:

1. Always eat burgers and sandwiches open-faced, throwing away the top slice of bread or bun.

2. Use, at most, one-third of the salad dressing normally provided in a sachet. There is far more than you would ever need, and adds unnecessary calories and salt to your meal. Choose the light or vinaigrette dressings over creamy ones.

Here is a more detailed rundown on your best choices at some of the larger fast-food chains:

SUBWAY
This chain has been a pacesetter in the fast-food industry by reducing fat and calories in its meals. Subway's 6-inch/6 g fat subs are your best choices; have them whole wheat or honey oat bread. Just be careful not to load on those high-fat/-calorie extras such as cheese, bacon, mayo and high-sugar sauces. Mr. Sub and other sandwich chains are following Subway's lead.

MCDONALD'S
McDonald's grilled chicken salads are a good bet along with a low-fat dressing. You can even go for a Fruit 'n' Yogurt Parfait dessert (hold the granola).

BURGER KING
Burger King's grilled chicken salads or chicken sandwich with garden salad are your best options. You may also consider a BK Veggie Burger (without mayo) and a garden salad.

WENDY'S
The Grilled Chicken Go Wrap is about your only alternative though you might consider a large chili with side salad. Their chicken salads are to be avoided as they are high in fat and sodium.

PIZZA HUT
Normally I recommend avoiding pizza restaurants so I am delighted to see that Pizza Hut has made a real effort to

improve its offerings. Your best bet is Thin 'N Crispy Pizzas and Fit 'N' Delicious Pizzas (2 slices maximum) plus garden salads and light dressings.

TACO BELL

Taco Bell's line of Fresco tacos are acceptable green-light choices, but are very high in sodium. Steer clear of the rest of the menu except the side salads.

KFC

Until KFC adopts grilled, as opposed to fried, chicken as they have in the U.S., it's a place to avoid.

RESTAURANTS

As it's almost impossible to list restaurants by name because of the regional nature of many chains, I thought it might be helpful if I provided you with a quick rundown on different types of restaurants instead.

FAMILY RESTAURANTS

This is a fast-growing segment of the restaurant business, which offers a very wide choice of foods and good value for a family eating out.

Though there are a few national chains such as Swiss Chalet, most are local operations. It would therefore be physically impossible to break out individual restaurants in the space available. However, the one overriding caution with these restaurants is portion size. Many serving sizes are large enough for two people. On a recent road trip, my wife and I found we could split many, if not most, of the courses and still come away satisfied. Also, ask if they can hold the cheese, which some restaurants add unnecessarily to many non-Asian dishes. You don't need those extra calories. If you are watchful, you can easily find many green-light alternatives to suit all the family.

The top-ten dining tips listed at the end of this chapter are particularly applicable to family restaurants.

ALL-YOU-CAN-EAT BUFFETS

This can be your worst or best option depending on your level of self-control. It's best to do a quick reconnaissance of the whole buffet before you start to fill your plate. This way you can pick out your best green-light choices ahead of time. Also start with a salad and a glass of water. All personality groups should review specific content set out in Chapter 7.

ITALIAN

I suggest you start with a good bean and vegetable soup, such as minestrone. For the main course your best option is grilled, roasted or braised fish, chicken or veal. You may order pasta as a side dish if you wish, but no cream sauces—you'll be better off with an extra serving of vegetables.

GREEK

Grilled or baked seafood is an excellent choice, as well as classic chicken souvlaki. Just watch your serving sizes. Instead of the potatoes, which are frequently served along with rice, order double vegetables. It is essential that you ask for both your salad dressing and feta to be served on the side.

CHINESE

This type of food can present some real challenges. Much of it is deep-fried with sweet sauces. Sodium levels are usually astronomic and the rice is glutinous and red-light (short-grain rice has a much higher G.I. than long-grain rice such as basmati). Though you can make do with steamed or stir-fried vegetables, it's probably not worth the effort. Chinese restaurants are my last resort when eating out.

INDIAN/SOUTH ASIAN

This is one of your best restaurant choices because of the cuisine's focus on vegetables, legumes, lentils and long-grain rice. Servings of meat, poultry or fish tend to be modest. However, ensure that the food is not fried, particularly not in "ghee" or clarified butter, which is a highly saturated fat. Also, be cautious with the side dishes such as mangoes/papayas, raisins and coconut slices as they have a high G.I. and can pack a lot of calories.

MEXICAN/LATIN AMERICAN

Tex-Mex dishes can be heavy on cheese, refried beans and sour cream, which are all red-light. Your best bet is to look for grilled seafood, chicken or meat, as well as dishes made with beans (not refried). Vegetable-based soups such as gazpacho are an excellent choice.

THAI

Thai restaurants tend to be heavy on red-light sauces, often using full-fat coconut milk. Here, it's best to stick with a starter such as lemongrass soup, green mango salad, or mussels in a lemongrass broth. Follow this with a Thai beef salad or stir-fry with chicken and vegetables. Skip the peanut sauce.

JAPANESE

This is a good green-light choice once you get beyond the sushi and tempura. Sushi is red-light because of the glutinous rice in it. Order the sashimi instead. Watch the quantity of soy sauce, which should be considered liquid salt! The beef and vegetable stir-fries and grilled fish are excellent choices. You might try nabemono, a healthy fondue with broth, rather than oil, as the cooking medium.

If you are dining in a group you might not have any say in the choice of restaurant. In that case, a little planning and some careful choices can help:

TOP-TEN DINING TIPS

Regardless of the type of restaurant you are dining in, the following ten tips will go a long way to ensure that you eat well while watching your waistline.

1. If possible, just before you go out, have a small bowl of high-fibre, green-light cold cereal (such as All-Bran) with skim milk and sweetener. I often add a couple of spoonfuls of fat-free fruit yogurt. This will take the edge off your appetite and get some fibre into your digestive system, which will help reduce the G.I. of your upcoming meal.

2. Once seated in the restaurant, drink a glass of water. It will help you feel fuller.

3. Remember to eat slowly to allow your brain the time it needs to realize you are full. Put your fork down between mouthfuls and savour your meal.

4. Once the basket of rolls or bread—which you will ignore—has been passed around the table, ask the server to remove it. The longer it sits, the more tempted you will be to dig in.

5. Order a soup or salad first and tell the server you would like this as soon as possible. This will keep you from sitting hungry while others are filling up on bread. For soups, go for vegetable or bean-based, the chunkier the better. Avoid any that are cream-based, such as vichyssoise. For salads, the golden rule is to keep the dressing on the side so you can use a fraction of what the restaurant would normally pour over your greens. Avoid Caesar salads, which come predressed and often pack as many calories as a burger.

6. Since you probably won't get boiled small or new potatoes and can't always be sure of what kind of rice is being served, ask for a double serving of vegetables instead. I have yet to find a restaurant that won't oblige.

7. Stick with low-fat cuts of meat or poultry. If necessary, you can remove the skin. Duck is usually too high in fat. Fish and shellfish are excellent choices but shouldn't be

breaded or battered. Tempura is more fat and flour than filling. Remember that servings tend to be generous in restaurants, so eat only 4 to 6 ounces (the size of a pack of cards) and leave the rest. Entrée sharing is also becoming a popular option.

8. As with salads, ask for any sauces or gravies to be served on the side.

9. For dessert, fresh fruit and berries—without the ice cream—are your best choice. If you are hankering for something sweet, sprinkle on some sweetener from one of the packages designed for coffee/tea. Most other desserts are a dietary disaster. My advice is to avoid dessert. If a birthday cake is being passed around, share your piece with someone. A couple of forkfuls with your decaf coffee should get you off the hook with minimal dietary damage!

10. Order only decaffeinated coffee. Skim-milk decaf cappuccino is our family's favourite choice.

Chapter Eleven
Staying Motivated

You wouldn't be human if you didn't feel your resolve starting to waver from time to time. It frequently has nothing to do with your diet but is related to other family, work or unrelated health stressors in your life. Plan how to maintain this motivation during those times when you feel you are not making enough progress or your stress levels become overwhelming. There are a number of things you can do to encourage yourself to keep going.

1. BODY IMAGE

You want to look better. Weight loss boosts self-esteem and confidence for women in particular. It's amazing the difference the loss of just a few pounds can make, not only in how you look in your clothes, but also to how you feel about yourself. For the Eater with Self-Esteem Issues, it is important to remember that the link between how you look and how you feel is critical. It is not superficial to want to look better, so stay with it—you deserve to feel happier with yourself.

2. ENERGY

Though body image doesn't appear to be a primary motivator for men, physical capability, strength and energy can be.

Being overweight means you have more pounds to carry around, which translates into flagging energy levels; sore back, hips and knees; and decreased mobility. The problem is that we don't realize what weight actually weighs. As suggested earlier, take a shopping bag and fill it up some water bottles to a weight of, say, 20 pounds (use bathroom scales) and carry it up and down two flights of stairs. You'll be glad to put the bag down. Unfortunately, you cannot do that with the weight that is stored around your waist and hips! I simply have no idea how some people carry around 50 or more extra pounds all the time. I doubt if many of them could actually lift that weight!

3. HEALTH

What you weigh and what you eat affects your risk of heart disease, stroke, diabetes and most cancers. Eating the right foods can improve your health and increase your energy levels to help you lead a longer and more active life. Many readers have written to me about the importance of being an active participant in their children and grandchildren's lives. It's hard to find a better motivator than that. Keep reminding yourself that good health is the most important asset in life and staying with the program is your best chance to promote it.

4. PHYSICAL REMINDERS

Judging by the number of e-mails I receive from readers about digging out skinny tops and pants that they had tucked away at the back of the wardrobe, dropping sizes is a tremendous motivator for women. Most women would prefer to shop for clothes that flatter and show off their bodies rather than resort to camouflage. It's a powerful motivator to walk into a room and hear a friend ask "Have you lost weight? You look terrific!" I've sold more books based on word of mouth than any other marketing strategy.

Body image is an important motivator for women (unfortunately, less so for men) so try keeping a picture of an outfit you're going to buy when you reach your goal, or a photograph of a thinner you, where you will see it every day. One reader, who is blind, kept a picture in her mind's eye. She told me "I am using my beautiful red leather coat as the motivator for me. Last winter when I went to put it on, it was about two inches too small. I was not able to close the zipper. Now when I put the coat on, I am able to zip up the coat. Tight yes, but I know that I have made progress. What an incredible feeling. What motivation for me as I am determined to wear the coat this winter."

Slimming down boosts self-esteem and confidence, which in turn makes it easier to maintain your new eating habits. It's amazing the difference that the loss of just a few pounds can make—not only in how you look in your clothes, but also in how you feel about yourself.

5. YOUR ACHIEVEMENTS

Compare yourself now to where you were before you started the diet. How much weight have you lost? How many inches have dropped from around your waist? Add in your new energy and clothes and you will be amazed to see how far you have come. Going back to your old eating habits won't seem so tempting when you think how it will undermine all the good things that this new way of living has brought you so far.

6. THE SHOPPING BAG MOTIVATOR

I mentioned previously that people frequently don't realize how much weight actually weighs. I know it sounds crazy, but when people tell me they've lost only 20 pounds, I ask them to fill a couple of shopping bags with plastic bottles filled with 20 pounds of water and carry them up and down the stairs a few times. Everyone is always glad to put the bags down. So the next time you're feeling uninspired, fill a shopping bag or two with bottles filled with water that equal the weight you've lost so far and carry them up and down a flight of stairs three times. You'll be amazed at what you've lost, and you'll be relieved to put the bags down. You couldn't have put that weight down when you started the program. This is dramatically demonstrated in a letter I received from Kathy:

I couldn't find bottles to fill to make 40 lbs, so I went to the grocery store. I was drawn to the potato aisle. There were 20 lb bags of potatoes, so I picked up two of these and they were so heavy, I felt a pressure right in the middle of my chest.

I thought, wow, I carried all that around with me every day . . . I tried to walk with them and I got tired after only fifteen steps. I'd die if I was to carry these up and down a flight of stairs.

I had a hard time breathing after this little test. What I decided was that it's not worth carrying all that weight around. I like my lighter body and I'm going to keep working on it to keep it this way.

7. GET SUPPORT

Buddy up with friends, a spouse or family members who are trying to lose weight. They will give you a sense of camaraderie and encouragement as you strive for your goal, and you can turn to them for support when you need it.

"Nothing succeeds like success" may sound like an overworked cliché, but as a motivator it is second to none. Keep a tally of your successes and always keep them in front of you—especially at those times when the spirit weakens, as it inevitably will. A weight-loss graph and/or plastic bottles are both excellent visual ways of doing this.

There are a couple of occasions when motivation becomes particularly important; namely, when you hit a weight-loss plateau or when you fall off the wagon. Here are some suggestions for dealing with these two inevitable challenges.

REACHING A PLATEAU

After diligently eating the green-light way and losing weight steadily for successive weeks, it is difficult to accept a break in that pattern. Unfair as it may be, it is inevitable. Weight loss never occurs in a straight line, but always in a series of steps or plateaus.

Plateaus are difficult for all personality traits. Controllers will worry and believe they are not being careful or rigid enough; they will look for more rules or give up because they find keeping to a diet boring and exhausting. Impulsive Eaters and Procrastinators, who need instant and frequent gratification, will feel frustrated and want to quit.

There are a couple of physical factors that influence plateaus. For women, hormonal shifts triggered by your monthly cycle or by menopause cause the body to retain fluid. This is nearly always a temporary state. As your hormones shift back to their previous levels, so will your fluids.

The other most common cause is "portion creep" as a weight-loss plateau can occur when you have let your guard down and allowed your portion or serving size to increase. This is easy to do. You have watched the pounds steadily drop off and now, not surprisingly, complacency can set in. A useful tool in keeping yourself on track is to divide your plate into three sections (see page 26); half the plate should consist of at least two vegetables; one-quarter should consist of a protein (meat, fish or tofu); and the remaining quarter can consist of rice, potatoes or pasta. And remember to use smaller lunch-sized plates instead of oversized dinner plates.

Since hormonal shifts and complacency can cause your weight to fluctuate significantly from day to day, I suggest you restrict your weigh-in to once a week or even once a month. Then you can avoid the disappointment of the short-term aberrations and focus on your long-term success. One reader wrote to me and said that she had become very frustrated with the daily variations in weight and decided to weigh herself once a month. She said that there was not a single month in the past eighteen months when she had not lost some weight and her frustration level had dropped significantly.

When playing the averages, patience is a virtue! Just keep on the green-light track and the weight will continue to come off. Some readers wonder why they sometimes seem to be losing inches but not pounds, and sometimes pounds but not inches. Remember, everyone is different, and weight loss doesn't ever happen in a straight line; eventually both the inches and pounds will come off—guaranteed!

So don't let a disappointment on the scale get you down. Nothing is quite as frustrating as hitting a weight-loss plateau. But if you hang in there and don't use food to console yourself, you will reach your weight-loss target.

FALLING OFF THE WAGON

Like a weight-loss plateau, falling off the wagon is bound to happen sooner or later. And while I don't encourage it, it's acceptable as long as it's the exception and not the rule. The diet isn't meant to be a straitjacket, after all. If you do your best to eat the green-light way 90 percent of the time, you will still lose weight. The odd lapse, at worst, will delay you by a week or two from reaching your target weight. So don't be too hard on yourself; just get right back on the plan with the next meal. Some people make the mistake of feeling so bad about a slip-up that they just give up. But you should anticipate that you will fall off the wagon from time to time. The best way to handle it is to learn why it happened and decide how you will handle the situation next time. By now you have the knowledge and tools to do just that.

For the Impulsive Eater and Procrastinator, here is another reason to quit: "See, I can't resist temptation so I might as well give up and admit defeat." Review your sections in Chapter 7 on changing behaviours—and keep going!"

Although most people find that their cravings diminish after few weeks on the G.I. Diet, because of the levelling effects green-light eating has on blood sugar levels, there will be times when a craving will surface. Here's how to handle the situation:

1. Try to distract yourself with an activity. Call a friend, fold a basket of laundry, take out the garbage or just go for a walk. Frequently, the craving will pass.

2. If you still have the craving, pinpoint the flavour that you want and find a green-light food that has it. For example, if you want something sweet and creamy, try low-fat yogurt or ice cream with no added sugar. If you want something salty, have a couple of olives or a dill pickle, or some hummus with veggies. If it's chocolate you crave, try half a chocolate-flavoured high-protein bar or a mug of instant light hot chocolate. There are many green-light versions of the foods we normally reach for when a craving strikes.

3. Sometimes nothing but a piece of chocolate or a spoonful of peanut butter will do. If this is the case, have a *small* portion and really enjoy it. Eat it slowly and savour the experience. Chalk it up to that 10 percent leeway you're allowed on the G.I Diet. Just make sure you're staying green-light 90 percent of the time.

This 10 percent wiggle room gives you permission to enjoy that extra serving or occasional drink. It is meant to help you stay with the program, so use it wisely.

Chapter Twelve
Exercise

Earlier in the book, I suggested that weight loss was 90 percent diet and 10 percent exercise, even though exercise is essential for weight maintenance and a healthy lifestyle.

To recap, there are two principal reasons exercise is not as efficient as diet when you are trying to lose weight. First, it requires a huge amount of effort to burn off those pounds. Take a good look at the table below. I doubt if many of you would be motivated, yet alone physically able, to lose weight this way.

effort required to lose 1 lb of fat		
	130-lb person	**160-lb person**
Walking (4 mph–brisk)	53 miles/85 km	42 miles/67 km
Running (8 min/mile)	36 miles/58 km	29 miles/46 km
Cycling (12–14 mph)	96 miles/154 km	79 miles/127 km
Sex (moderate effort)	79 times	64 times

I'm sure many of you have tried a treadmill or exercise bike some time in your life and have been amazed at how much effort it takes to burn off even 200 calories.

As one pound of fat contains 3,600 calories, you can see why taking the dog for a walk around the block or washing the car has little or no impact on losing weight. Obviously, any exercise is better than none, as it all helps to burn extra calories. Just don't expect it to have any significant impact during the weight-loss phase.

The second reason I recommend diet rather than exercise during the weight-loss period is the difficulty obese people—those with a BMI of 30 and over—have in physical movement. Quite frankly, I am astonished that many of the big people I have met can actually support their weight. The stress on joints and back carrying an additional 80 to 100 pounds or more is absolutely enormous. Most people couldn't even lift that weight, yet alone carry it around all the time. This puts a serious limitation on what overweight people can do to exercise, even if they wanted to.

However, if you are nearing your weight-loss goals, this is the time to consider getting more active. The upside of exercise is that, *over the long term,* it can help you maintain or accelerate your weight loss, as well as contribute significantly to your health by reducing your risk of heart disease, stroke, diabetes and osteoporosis. It will also help maintain your muscle mass and tone.

Exercise should become an important consideration for those of you moving from being "obese" to "overweight." Most of you are now better able to exercise as you have less weight to carry around, and you should also be experiencing an increase in your energy level.

Those of you who decide to do something are frequently lured by fitness clubs that promise a dream body if only you'll sign up. Disappointment is the usual outcome. A principal reason for the very high membership turnover in fitness clubs is their failure to deliver on their weight-loss promises. Those clubs that emphasize diet as a core component of their program are usually the ones that are more successful.

The simplest activity is walking. This doesn't require any special equipment or gym membership, and can be done at virtually any time of the day or year. If you still find it difficult to walk any distance, then an indoor stationary bike is a good investment. The reclining-position bikes are probably easier on your joints as your weight load is spread over a greater area.

These are relatively inexpensive and available through many large retail chains such as Canadian Tire. Otherwise, join a gym and use the heavy-duty equipment, particularly if your BMI is 30 plus.

Walking thirty minutes a day, seven days a week, should be your target. If you add an hour-long walk on the weekend, you can take a day off during the week. As mentioned before, we're talking about brisk walking—not speed walking or ambling. It must increase your heart and breathing rate, but never exercise to the point where you cannot find the breath to converse with a partner.

You don't need any special clothing or equipment except a pair of comfortable cushioned shoes or sneakers. Walking is rarely boring since you can keep changing routes and watch the world go by as you exercise. Walk with a friend for company and mutual support, or go solo and commune with nature and your own thoughts. I do my best thinking of the day on my morning walk. This is not surprising when you realize how much extra oxygen-fresh blood is pumping through your brain.

A great idea is to incorporate walking into your daily commute to work. I got off the bus two stops early on my way to and from work. Those two stops are equal to about 2 kilometres, so I'm walking about 4 kilometres per day! If you drive to work, try parking your car about 2 kilometres away and walk to your job. You may even find cheaper parking farther out.

This investment of an extra 10 to 15 minutes a day each way will pay real dividends for maintaining your weight and health.

I used to do this and found that far from being a drag or inconvenience, I actually looked forward to my "two stops short" walk each day. It helped get me going in the morning and gave me time to reflect on my day with no phones or people crowding me. In the evening, it was a chance to wind down and relax. It required some effort for the first week, but quickly became routine for my last three years at the Heart and Stroke Foundation.

In summary then, exercise is of more limited value during the relatively short time when you are actually losing weight. It is, however, a critical factor in maintaining your weight and health for the rest of your life. Believe it or not, exercise can become addictive and I know that I become irritable and edgy if I'm not getting my daily exercise fix—or so my wife Ruth tells me!

Though I have focused on aerobic exercise, the sort of exercise that increases your heart rate, there are several other important considerations regarding exercise that you should be considering. The most important of these are resistance exercises, which are aimed at strengthening your muscles.

An insidious and silent change that takes place as we age is the loss or thinning of muscle mass. This is a process that starts in our twenties, and by middle age most people have lost around 15 percent of their muscle mass. From middle age onward the rate of muscle loss escalates quickly.

So why does this loss matter? First, you risk becoming frail as you lack muscle to move and stabilize your body. Without strong muscles in legs and hips, women in particular are at significant risk of a debilitating fall and broken bones or worse.

Second, less muscle means a lower metabolic rate. Muscles are the principal consumer of your body's energy (calories); so the less muscle, the fewer calories you burn and we all know where those surplus calories go: fat replaces muscle. Fat, conversely, burns few calories.

However, all is not lost. There are a couple of things you can do to help offset this decline and raise your metabolic rate.

The first is to make sure you are getting adequate protein in your diet. The best sources of lean protein are chicken/turkey (skinless), fish, eggs (liquid), lean meats, low-fat dairy, soy and legumes (beans). Ideally every snack and certainly every meal should have some protein content. A further benefit of protein is that it slows the digestion and therefore effectively lowers the G.I. of the meal.

The second offset is exercise. I do not mean aerobic exercise (the type of exercise that increases your heart rate such as walking or jogging) but, rather, resistance exercises. These work muscles against some form of resistance; weights and elastic bands are the two most popular. These are the only exercises that build muscle mass. I'm sure most of you associate weights with an image of overmuscled men sweating and grunting with giant barbells. Don't panic, the reality is far less daunting—even a can of soup can act as a weight.

I don't propose to detail an exact program here, as everyone's needs and budgets are different. Rather, I recommend going to the U.S. Government Center for Disease Control and Prevention site (www.CDC.gov/physicalactivity). Click on "Growing Stronger—Strength Training for Older Adults"; and on that page click "Exercises." This is an excellent site that demonstrates how to do the various exercises—and it's free!

Boosting your protein intake and adding a few minutes of simple resistance exercises three times a week will go a long way toward stabilizing your muscle loss—and if you are diligent, actually rebuilding some of that loss. You will be less frail and less prone to falling, as well as able to consume more calories. Remember, muscles consume calories even when they are at rest and even when sleeping.

Many of you will be muttering by now about how this would all sound fine if we lived in California, but get real, this is Canada; you can't do many of these activities for half the year.

The alternative is either a home gym or a fitness club. The latter is an easy option these days in most larger communities. Clubs offer not only a wide range of sophisticated equipment, but also mutual support from friends and expert advice from staff.

If a fitness club isn't convenient or those Lycra-clad young things make you uncomfortable, the simple alternative is to exercise at home. As mentioned earlier, the best and least expensive equipment is a stationary exercise bike.

You can easily pay into the thousands for a bike with all the fancy trimmings—one that is designed for use in a fitness club—but in reality a $250 to $350 machine will work fine. Just be sure it has smooth, adjustable tension and proper seat height, then plug in a movie or your favourite soap and get pedalling. You'll be amazed how quickly the minutes fly by. I've frequently gone way over my scheduled time as I've become immersed in the screen action! Twenty minutes on the bike will give you the same calorie consumption as thirty minutes of brisk walking.

If biking is not for you, try a treadmill. These can be expensive, and beware the lower-end models that cannot take the pounding. Expect to pay about $700 to $1,000, and ensure that the incline of the track can be raised and lowered for a better workout.

GETTING STARTED

Now that you're convinced exercise is for you, how do you go about getting started?

1. Select an exercise that suits you. The fastest way to abandon an exercise program is to do something you don't enjoy. It is best to select an exercise that uses the largest muscle groups, that is, the legs, abdominals and lower back. These burn more calories because of their sheer size. Walking and biking are excellent choices.
2. Get support from family and friends. If possible, find a like-minded buddy to exercise with you.
3. Set goals and keep a record. Put it on the fridge or in the bathroom.
4. Check with your doctor to ensure that he/she supports your plan.

Chapter Thirteen
Health

Food impacts our health in two ways. First, your choice of foods and the quantity you consume will be key determinants in how much you weigh. And the connection between being overweight and being at increased risk for diseases such as heart disease, stroke and diabetes is well established.

Second, the types of protein, fat and carbohydrates you consume can determine your risk level for heart disease, stroke, diabetes, prostate and colon cancers and Alzheimer's. Making the right food choices has been the principal theme of *The G.I. Diet*. In this chapter we will examine the role of diet in preventing diseases.

Foods are, in effect, drugs. They have a powerful influence on our health, well-being and emotional state. We take in food four or five times a day, usually with more thought for taste than for nutritional value. It would be incomprehensible to take drugs on the same basis.

The right foods can help you maintain your health, extend your lifespan, give you more energy, and make you feel good and sleep better. Couple that with exercise and you are doing all you can to keep healthy, fit and alert. The rest is a matter of genes and luck.

We'll now examine the role of diet and exercise in preventing diseases.

HEART DISEASE AND STROKE

Given that I was the president of the Heart and Stroke Foundation of Ontario for fifteen years, it is hardly surprising that I'm starting with these diseases. However, there is a more important reason: heart disease and stroke account for 35 percent of North American deaths. Remarkably, this is evidence of progress. When I first joined the foundation, the figure was close to 50 percent.

This is a good news, bad news story. The good news is that advances in surgery, drug therapies and emergency services have saved many lives. The bad news is that twice as many deaths could have been averted if only we had reduced our weight, exercised regularly and quit smoking. Though the smoking rate for adults has dropped sharply (unfortunately, we cannot say the same for teens), we are eating more and exercising less, leading inevitably to a more obese and unhealthy population. It's been calculated that if we led even a moderate lifestyle, we could halve the carnage from these diseases. Though heart disease, like most cancers, is primarily a disease of old age, nearly half of those who suffer heart attacks are under the age of sixty-five.

A familiar refrain that I have heard many times is, "Why worry? If I have a heart attack, today's medicine will save me." It might well save you from immediate death, but what most people do not realize is that the heart is permanently damaged after an attack. The heart cannot repair itself because its cells do not reproduce. (Ever wonder why you cannot get cancer of the heart? That's the reason.) After the damage sustained during a heart attack, the heart has to work harder to compensate—but it never can. It slowly degenerates under this stress, and patients finally "drown" as blood circulation fails and the lungs fill with liquid. Congestive heart failure is a dreadful way to die, so make sure you do everything you can to avoid having a heart attack in the first place.

For many years, heart attacks were considered to be a man's domain, which still is more often than not the case for men under the age of fifty, but after that it becomes a common cause for both men *and* women.

With regard to diet, the simple fact is that the fatter you are, the more likely it is you will suffer a heart attack or stroke. The two key factors that link heart disease and stroke to diet are cholesterol and hypertension (high blood pressure). I promised at the beginning of this book that I was not going to dwell on the complexities of the science of nutrition; it's the outcome of this science that's important. However, a little science is helpful to understand the role and importance of both hypertension and cholesterol.

Hypertension is the harbinger of both heart disease and stroke. High blood pressure puts more stress on the arterial system and causes it to age and deteriorate more rapidly, ultimately leading to arterial damage, blood clots, and heart attack or stroke. Excess weight has a major bearing on high blood pressure. A recent Canadian study found that obese adults, aged eighteen to fifty-five, had a five to thirteen times greater risk of hypertension. A further study demonstrated that a lower-fat diet coupled with a major increase in the consumption of fruits and vegetables (eight to ten servings a day) lowered blood pressure. The moral: lose weight and eat more fruits and vegetables to help reduce your blood pressure levels. In other words, adopt the G.I. Diet.

Cholesterol is essential to your body's metabolism. However, high cholesterol is a problem as it's the key ingredient in the plaque that can build up in your arteries, eventually cutting off the blood supply to your heart (causing heart attack) or your brain (leading to stroke). To make things more complicated, there are two forms of cholesterol: HDL (good) cholesterol and LDL (bad) cholesterol. The idea is to boost the HDL level while depressing the LDL level. (Remember it this way: HDL is Heart's Delight Level and LDL is Leads to Death Level.)

The villain in raising LDL levels is saturated fat, which is usually solid at room temperature and is found primarily in meat and whole milk and food products. Conversely, polyunsaturated and monounsaturated fats not only lower LDL levels but actually boost HDL. The moral: make sure some fat is included in your diet, but make sure it's the right fat. (Refer to chapter 1 for the complete rundown on fat.)

DIABETES

Diabetes is the kissing cousin of heart disease in that more people die from heart complications arising from diabetes than from diabetes alone. And diabetes rates are skyrocketing: they are expected to double in the next ten years. The latest U.S. figures are staggering: thirty-seven percent of adults are diagnosed as either diabetic or pre-diabetic. I repeat, thirty-seven percent.

The principal causes of the most common form of diabetes, Type 2, are obesity and lack of exercise, and the current epidemic is strongly correlated to the obesity trend. Foods with a low G.I., which release sugar more slowly into the bloodstream, appear to play a major role in helping diabetics control their disease. Thus the G.I. Diet provides an opportunity both to lose weight—the principal cause of diabetes—and to assist in the management of the symptoms. In their magazine *Dialogue*, the Canadian Diabetes Association selected the G.I. Diet as their diet of choice. Because protein and fat have an impact on food's G.I. ratings, diabetics should be particularly careful about eating the right balance of green-light proteins, carbohydrates and fats at every meal and snack. Prevention, however, is far preferable, so get right into your G.I. Diet program and get those pounds off.

Evidence of the G.I. Diet's effectiveness in reducing blood sugar levels is featured in my recent book *The G.I. Diet Diabetes Clinic*, which was based on an e-clinic I conducted with thirty-eight diabetics. Participants were able to reduce their A1C levels by an average of 15 percent in just three months.

CANCER

In one of the largest studies to date, British scientists pooled information from 141 studies on twenty different cancers. They found conclusive evidence that obesity was replacing smoking as the number-one risk factor for cancer. They demonstrated a depressing series of links between being overweight and

- Esophagal, thyroid, kidney and colon cancers; multiple myeloma, leukemia and non-Hodgkin's lymphoma in both sexes.
- Rectal cancer and malignant melanoma in men.
- Gallbladder, pancreatic, endometrial cancers and postmenopausal breast cancer in women.

A recent global report by the American Institute for Cancer Research concluded that 30 to 40 percent of cancers are directly linked to dietary choices. Its key recommendation is that individuals should choose a diet that includes a variety of vegetables, fruit and grains and is low in saturated fat—the G.I. Diet in a nutshell.

ALZHEIMER'S DISEASE

As with cancer, there is increasing evidence linking certain dementias, particularly Alzheimer's, with fat intake. A recent U.S. study showed a 40 percent increase in Alzheimer's disease for those who ate a diet high in saturated fat.

ABDOMINAL FAT

The most alarming medical news about abdominal fat is that it is not, as previously thought, a passive accumulator of energy reserves and extra baggage. Rather it is an active, living part of your body. Once it has formed sufficient mass, it behaves like any other organ such as the liver, heart or kidney, except that it pumps out a dangerous combination of free fatty acids and proteins. This causes out-of-control cell proliferation, which is directly associated with the growth of malignant cancer tumours. It also creates inflammation, which is linked to atherosclerosis, the principal cause of heart disease and stroke. And if that weren't bad enough, fat tissues also increase insulin resistance, leading to Type 2 diabetes.

The fact is that abdominal fat has many of the characteristics of a huge tumour—and that thought may help encourage any fence-sitters out there to start doing something about their weight.

SUPPLEMENTS

Providing you are eating the green-light way, you are receiving all the nutrients necessary for a healthy life. There are, however, two important exceptions:

Vitamin D

Vitamin D is known as the sunshine vitamin for very good reason. It is synthesized by the interaction of sunlight on our skin. Its incidence in food is very limited and is primarily confined to fatty fish such as salmon or in fortified milk products. This vitamin is particularly important in reducing your risk for cancer, heart disease and osteoporosis. The problem is that for Canadians sunshine is a scarce commodity in winter, and since we should be lathered in sunscreen during our brief summer, we are unable to capitalize on this vitamin's self-generation.

Most authorities now recommend a daily supplement of 1000 I.U. of this inexpensive vitamin.

Fish Oil

There is one oil in particular that has been found to have significant positive health benefits, particularly for your heart. The oil is called omega-3, which is a fatty acid found primarily in coldwater fish, salmon in particular, as well as a modest amount in canola and flaxseed. As most of us are unlikely to consume salmon on a daily basis, salmon oil is available in capsule form in any pharmacy.

KNEE AND HIP REPLACEMENT

Finally, there is the issue of joint degeneration caused by excessive weight loading. Just recently the Canadian Institute of Health published a survey of knee and hip replacements performed in Canada in 2004/5. It showed that not only had the number of operations nearly doubled over the past ten years, but that the overweight and obese patient accounted for a startling 87 percent of knee replacements and 74 percent of hip. Some 54 percent of the knee-replacement patients were obese, though this group accounted for only 23 percent of the population. Interestingly, 60 percent of patients were women whose smaller bone structure makes them more vulnerable to stress from extra weight.

So if you want to reduce your risk of incurring these leading killer diseases—heart disease, stroke, diabetes, hypertension and cancer—and keep your joints intact—then stay with the program. I can't think of a better motivator.

Appendix I
Complete G.I. Diet Food Guide

	RED	YELLOW	GREEN
BEANS			
	Baked beans with pork	Chili	Baked beans (low-fat)
	Broad	Kidney beans (canned)	Black beans
	Refried	Lentils (canned)	Black-eyed peas
			Butter beans
			Cannellini
			Chickpeas/garbanzo
			Italian
			Kidney
			Lentils
			Lima
			Mung
			Navy
			Pigeon
			Pinto
			Refried (low-fat)
			Romano
			Soybeans
			Split peas
BEVERAGES			
	Alcoholic drinks*	Diet soft drinks (caffeinated)	Bottled water
	Coconut milk	Milk (1%)	Club soda
	Fruit drinks	Most unsweetened juice	Decaffeinated coffee (with skim milk, no sugar)

*Limit serving size (see page 45).

	RED	YELLOW	GREEN
	Milk (whole or 2%)	Red wine**	Diet soft drinks (no caffeine)
	Regular coffee	Vegetable juices	Herbal tea
	Regular soft drinks	Coconut milk (low-fat)	Light instant chocolate
	Rice milk		Milk (skim)
	Sweetened juice		Soy milk (plain, low-fat)
	Watermelon juice		Tea (with skim milk, no sugar)

BREADS

	RED	YELLOW	GREEN
	Bagels	Crispbreads (with fibres)	Crispbreads (with high fibre, e.g., Wasa Fibre)*
	Baguette/Croissants	Pita (whole wheat)	Pita (high fibre)
	Cake/Cookies	Tortillas (whole wheat)	Whole-grain, high-fibre breads (min. 3 g fibre per slice)*
	Cornbread	Whole-grain breads	
	Crispbreads (regular)		
	Croutons		
	English muffins		
	Hamburger buns		
	Hot dog buns		
	Kaiser rolls		
	Melba toast		
	Muffins/Doughnuts		
	Pancakes/Waffles		
	Pizza		
	Stuffing		
	Tortillas		
	White bread		

CEREALS

	RED	YELLOW	GREEN
	All cold cereals except those listed as yellow- or green-light	Kashi Good Friends	100% bran
	Cereal/Granola bars	Shredded Wheat Bran	All-Bran

*Limit serving size (see page 25).
**Limit serving size (see page 45).

184

	RED	YELLOW	GREEN
	Granola		Bran Buds
	Grits		Cold cereals with minimum 10 g fibre per serving
	Muesli (commercial)		Fibre 1
			Fibre First
			Kashi Go Lean
			Kashi Go Lean Crunch
			Oat Bran
			Porridge (large-flake or steel cut oats)
			Red River

CEREAL/GRAINS

	RED	YELLOW	GREEN
	Amaranth	Cornstarch	Arrowroot flour
	Almond flour	Spelt	Barley
	Couscous	Whole wheat	Bran (wheat/oat)
	Millet	Couscous	Buckwheat
	Polenta	Oatmeal (instant/quick cook)	Bulgar
	Rice (short-grain, white, instant)		Gram flour
	Rice cakes		Kamut
	Rice noodles		Kasha (not puffed)
	White flour		Quinoa
			Rice (basmati, wild, brown, long-grain)
			Wheat berries
			Wheat germ
			Whole wheat flour

CONDIMENTS/SEASONINGS

	RED	YELLOW	GREEN
	BBQ sauce	Mayonnaise (light)	Capers
	Croutons		Chili powder
	Honey mustard		Extracts (vanilla, etc.)
	Ketchup		Garlic
	Mayonnaise		Gravy mix (maximum 20 calories per ¼-cup serving)

	RED	YELLOW	GREEN
	Relish		Herbs
	Steak sauce		Horseradish
	Tartar sauce		Hummus
			Mayonnaise (fat-free)
			Mustard
			Salsa (no added sugar)
			Sauerkraut
			Soy sauce (low sodium)
			Spices
			Teriyaki sauce
			Vinaigrette
			Vinegar (all types)
			Worcestershire sauce
DAIRY			
	Almond milk	Cheese (low-fat)	Buttermilk
	Cheese	Cream cheese (light)	Cheese (extra low-fat)
	Chocolate milk	Ice cream (low-fat)	Cottage cheese (1% or fat-free)
	Coconut milk	Milk (1%)	Cream cheese (fat-free)
	Cottage cheese (whole or 2%)	Sour cream (light)	Extra low-fat cheese (e.g., Laughing Cow Light, Boursin Light)
	Cream	Yogurt (low-fat, with sugar)	Frozen yogurt 1/2 cup (low-fat)
	Cream cheese		Flavoured yogurt (non-fat with sweetener)
	Evaporated milk		Ice cream (1/2 cup, low-fat and no added sugar)
	Goat milk		Milk (skim)
	Ice cream		Sour cream (1% or less)
	Milk (whole or 2%)		Soy milk (plain, low-fat)
	Rice milk		Soy cheese (low-fat)

	RED	YELLOW	GREEN
	Sour cream		Whey protein powder
	Yogurt (whole or 2%)		
FATS			
	Butter	100% nut butters	Almonds*
	Coconut oil	100% peanut butter	Canola oil*/seed
	Hard margarine	Corn oil	Cashews*
	Lard	Mayonnaise (light)	Flax seed
	Mayonnaise	Nuts (except those listed green-light)	Hazelnuts*
	Palm oil	Peanuts	Macadamia nuts*
	Peanut butter (regular and light)	Peanut oil	Mayonnaise (fat-free)
	Salad dressings (regular)	Pecans	Olive oil*
	Tropical oils	Salad dressings (light)	Pistachios*
	Vegetable shortening	Sesame oil	Salad dressings (low-fat, low-sugar)
		Soft margarine (non-hydrogenated)	Soft margarine (non-hydrogenated, light)*
		Soy oil	Vegetable oil sprays
		Sunflower oil	Vinaigrette
		Vegetable oils	
FRUITS			
Fresh/ Frozen	Cantaloupe	Apricots	Apples
	Honeydew melon	Bananas	Avocado* (1/4)
	Kumquats	Custard apples	Blackberries
	Watermelon	Figs	Cherries
		Kiwi	Cranberries
		Mango	Grapefruit
		Papaya	Grapes
		Persimmon	Guavas
		Pineapple	Lemons
		Pomegranates	Nectarines
			Oranges (all varieties)

*Limit serving size (see page 25).

	RED	YELLOW	GREEN
			Peaches
			Plums
			Pears
			Raspberries
			Rhubarb
			Strawberries
Bottled, Canned and Dried	All canned fruit in syrup	Canned apricots in juice or water	Applesauce (without sugar)
	Applesauce containing sugar	Dried apricots*	Dried apples
	Most dried fruit** (including dates and raisins)	Dried cranberries*	Fruit spreads with fruit, not sugar as the main ingredient
	Prunes	Fruit cocktail in juice	Mandarin oranges
		Peaches/pears in syrup	Peaches/pears in juice or water

JUICES**

	RED	YELLOW	GREEN
	Fruit drinks	Apple (unsweetened)	
	Prune	Cranberry (unsweetened)	
	Sweetened juice	Grapefruit (unsweetened)	
	Watermelon	Orange (unsweetened)	
		Pear (unsweetened)	
		Pineapple (unsweetened)	
		Vegetable	

MEAT, POULTRY, FISH, EGGS AND MEAT SUBSTITUTES

	RED	YELLOW	GREEN
	Beef (brisket, short ribs)	Beef (sirloin steak, sirloin tip)	All fish and seafood, fresh, frozen or canned (in water)
	Bologna	Chicken/turkey leg (skinless)	Back bacon
	Breaded fish and seafood	Corned beef	Beef (top/eye round steak)
	Duck	Dried beef	Chicken breast (skinless)

*For baking, it is OK to use a modest amount of dried apricots or cranberries.
**Whenever possible, eat the fruit rather than drink its juice.

	RED	YELLOW	GREEN
	Goose	Fish canned in oil	Egg whites
	Ground beef (more than 10% fat)	Flank steak	Ground beef (extra lean)
	Hamburgers	Ground beef (lean)	Lean deli meats
	Hot dogs	Lamb (fore/leg shank, centre cut loin chop)	Liquid eggs (e.g., Break Free)
	Lamb (rack)	Pork (centre loin, fresh ham, shank, sirloin, top loin)	Moose
	Organ meats	Tofu (firm)	Pastrami (turkey)
	Pastrami (beef)	Turkey bacon	Pork tenderloin
	Pâté	Whole regular eggs (preferably omega-3)	Rabbit
	Pork (back ribs, blade, spare ribs)		Sashimi
	Regular bacon		Soy/Whey protein powder
	Salami		Soy cheese (low fat)
	Sausages		Tofu (soft)
	Sushi		Turkey breast (skinless)
			Turkey roll
			TVP (Textured Vegetable Protein)
			Veal
			Veggie burger
			Venison
PASTA			
	All canned pastas		Capellini
	Gnocchi		Fettuccine
	Macaroni and cheese		Macaroni
	Noodles (canned or instant)		Mung bean noodles
	Pasta filled with cheese or meat		Penne
	Rice noodles		Rigatoni
			Spaghetti/Linguine
			Vermicelli

	RED	YELLOW	GREEN
PASTA SAUCES			
	Alfredo	Basil pesto	Light sauces with vegetables (no added sugar, e.g., Healthy Choice)
	Sauces with added meat or cheese	Sun-dried tomato pesto	
	Sauces with added sugar or sucrose		
SNACKS			
	Bagels	Bananas	Almonds*
	Candy	Dark chocolate ** (70% cocoa)	Applesauce (unsweetened)
	Cookies	Ice cream (low-fat)	Canned peaches/ pears in juice or water
	Crackers	Nuts* (except those listed green-light)	Cottage cheese (1% or fat-free)
	Doughnuts	Popcorn (light, microwaveable)	Extra low-fat cheese (e.g., Laughing Cow Light, Boursin Light)
	Flavoured gelatin (all varieties)		Flavoured yogurt (non-fat with sweetener)
	French fries		Frozen yogurt 1/2 cup (low-fat)
	Ice cream		Hazelnuts*
	Melba toast		High protein bars**
	Muffins (commercial)		Ice cream (1/2 cup, low-fat and no added sugar)
	Popcorn (regular)		Macadamia nuts*
	Potato chips		Most fresh/frozen fruit
	Pretzels		Most fresh/frozen vegetables
	Pudding		Most seeds
	Raisins		Pickles
	Rice cakes/crackers		Soy nuts
	Sorbet		Sugar-free hard candies

*Limit serving size (see page 25).
**180-225 calorie bars, e.g., Zone or Balance Bars; 1/2 bar per serving.

	RED	YELLOW	GREEN
	Tortilla chips		
	Trail mix		
	White bread		
SOUPS			
	All cream-based soups	Canned chicken noodle	Chunky bean and vegetable soups (e.g., Campbell's Healthy Request, Healthy Choice)
	Canned black bean	Canned lentil	Homemade soups with green-light ingredients
	Canned green pea	Canned tomato	Miso soup
	Canned puréed vegetable		
	Canned split pea		
SPREADS AND PRESERVES			
	All products that have sugar as the first ingredient listed		Fruit spreads (with fruit, not sugar, as the first ingredient)
			Marmite
SUGAR AND SWEETENERS			
	Agave nectar	Fructose	Splenda
	Corn syrup	Sugar alcohols (eg. maltitol, xylitol)	Stevia
	Glucose		Sugar Twin
	Honey		Sugar Twin Brown
	Molasses		Sweet'N Low
	Sugar (all types)		
	Sugar Blend		
	Splenda Brown		
VEGETABLES (FRESH/FROZEN)			
	Broad beans	Artichokes	Alfalfa sprouts
	Coleslaw (commercial)	Beets	Asparagus
	French fries	Corn	Beans (green/wax)
	Hash browns	Potatoes (boiled)	Bell peppers
	Parsnips	Pumpkin	Bok choy
	Potatoes (instant)	Squash	Broccoli

	RED	YELLOW	GREEN
	Potatoes (mashed or baked)	Sweet potatoes	Brussels sprouts
	Rutabaga	Yams	Cabbage (all varieties)
	Turnip		Carrots
			Cauliflower
			Celery
			Collard greens
			Cucumbers
			Eggplant
			Fennel
			Garlic
			Hearts of palm
			Kale
			Kohlrabi
			Leeks
			Lettuce
			Mushrooms
			Mustard greens
			Okra
			Olives*
			Onions
			Peas
			Peppers (hot)
			Potatoes (boiled, small, preferably new)
			Radicchio
			Radishes
			Rapini
			Salad greens (all varieties)
			Snow peas
			Spinach
			Swiss chard
			Tomatoes
			Zucchini

*Limit serving size (see page 25).

192

Appendix II
G.I. Diet Shopping List

PANTRY	FRIDGE/FREEZER
BAKING/COOKING	**DAIRY**
Baking powder/soda	Buttermilk
Cocoa	Cottage cheese (1%)
Dried apricots	Ice cream (low-fat, no added sugar)
Sliced almonds	Milk (skim)
Wheat/oat bran	Sour cream (fat-free or 1%)
Whole wheat flour	Soy milk (plain, low-fat)
BEANS (CANNED)	Yogurt (nonfat with sugar substitute)
Baked beans (low-fat)	**FRUIT (FRESH / FROZEN)**
Mixed salad beans	Apples
Most varieties	Blackberries
Vegetarian chili	Blueberries
BREAD	Cherries
whole wheat 3 g fibre/slice	Grapefruit
CEREALS	Grapes
All-Bran	Lemons
Bran Buds	Limes
Fibre First	Oranges
Kashi Go Lean	Peaches
Oat/wheat bran	Pears

PANTRY	FRIDGE/FREEZER
Oatmeal (old-fashioned rolled oats)	Plums
DRINKS	Raspberries
Bottled water	Strawberries
Club soda	**MEAT/POULTRY/FISH/EGGS**
Decaffeinated coffee	All fish and seafood (no breading)
Diet soft drinks (caffeine free)	Chicken/Turkey breast (skinless)
Tea	Extra-lean ground beef
FATS/OILS	Lean deli-style ham/turkey/chicken
Almonds	Liquid eggs (Break Free/Omega Pro)
Canola oil	Pork tenderloin
Margarine (non-hydrogenated, light)	Veal
Mayonnaise (fat-free)	Meat substitutes (see Complete Food Listings)
Olive oil	**VEGETABLES**
Salad dressings (fat-free)	Asparagus
Vegetable oil spray	Beans (green/wax)
FRUIT (CANNED/BOTTLED)	Bell and hot peppers
Applesauce (no sugar)	Broccoli
Mandarin oranges	Cabbage
Peaches in juice or water	Carrots
Pears in juice or water	Cauliflower
	Celery

PANTRY	FRIDGE/FREEZER
	Cucumber
PASTA	Eggplant
Capellini	Leeks
Fettuccine	Lettuce
Macaroni	Mushrooms
Penne	Olives
Spaghetti	Onions
Vermicelli	Pickles
PASTA SAUCES (Vegetable-based only)	Potatoes (small, preferably new only)
Healthy Choice	Snow peas
Too Good To Be True	Spinach
RICE	Tomatoes
Basmati/long grain/wild	Zucchini
SEASONINGS	**SOUPS**
Flavoured vinegars/sauces	Healthy Choice
Spices/herbs	**SWEETENERS**
SNACKS	Splenda, Sweet'n Low,
Food bars (Zone/Balance)	Sugar Twin (and other sugar substitutes)

Appendix III
The Ten Golden G.I. Diet Rules

1. Eat three meals and three snacks every day. Don't skip meals—particularly breakfast.
2. Stick with green-light products only in Phase I.
3. When it comes to food, quantity is as important as quality. Shrink your usual portions, particularly of meat, pasta and rice.
4. Always ensure that each meal contains a measure of carbohydrates, protein and fat.
5. Eat at least three times more vegetables and fruit than usual.
6. Drink plenty of fluids, preferably water.
7. Stay 90 percent on the program and allow yourself 10 percent wiggle room. This diet is not a straitjacket.
8. Find a friend to join you for mutual support.
9. Set realistic goals. Try to lose an average of a pound a week and record your progress to reinforce your sense of achievement.
10. Try not to view this as a diet, but rather the basis of how you will eat for the rest of your life.

G.I. DIET WEEKLY WEIGHT/WAIST LOG

WEEK	DATE	WEIGHT	WAIST	COMMENTS
1.				
2.				
3.				
4.				
5.				
6.				
7.				
8.				
9.				
10.				
11.				
12.				
13.				
14.				
15.				
16.				
17.				
18.				
19.				
20.				

Acknowledgements

My thanks and deep appreciation to my friends at Random House Canada who took a flyer on a couple of relative unknowns, myself and the glycemic index, several years ago. I am particularly appreciative of the counsel and wise advice from Anne Collins, Vice President and Publisher, and for the warm and patient editing of Stacey Cameron and more recently, Pamela Murray. Thanks also go to Jennifer Shepherd, who masterminded the selling of international rights in twenty-three countries and seventeen languages around the world.

To my cheerleader, business adviser and agent, Bruce Westwood, who along with his additional right hand, Natasha Daneman, have been invaluable in extending the G.I. Diet program.

Finally to my wife and partner, Dr. Ruth Gallop, whose insight into personality and its impact on eating behaviours has added a valuable dimension to the book. Also for her encouragement and support, without which I doubt *The G.I. Diet* would have seen the light of day.

Index

and labels, 50
in "slow-release" foods, 12–13
Fibre First cereal, 28, 185
fish, 13, 25, 33, 36, 42, 46, 69, 92, 119–22, 161, 173, 181, 188, 189
    benefits of, 6, 42
    breaded or coated, 28, 42, 92, 162, 188
    charts, 33, 38,
    serving size, 25
    and vitamin D, 181
fish oil, 6, 181
flavonoids, 45, 56
flax seed, 6, 181, 187
flour, 7, 8, 185
food bars, 36
food charts
    breakfast, 28–29
    dinner, 39–41
    fats, 29, 34, 40, 187
    G.I. ratings (sample),10
    grain consumption, 8
    lunch, 33–35
    snacks, 37
food guide, 184–92
fructose, 51, 191
fruit cocktail, 28, 188
fruit drinks, 29, 45, 183, 188
fruit juices, 45
fruits, 12, 30. See also specific fruits
    better than fruit juices, 45
    charts, 28, 34, 39, 187–88
    as dessert, 43–44
    dried, 28, 29, 34, 40, 139, 140, 145, 146, 188
    fibre and citrus, 12
    fresh, 28, 34, 37, 39, 43, 46, 82, 94, 95, 97, 106, 147, 162,
    as snacks, 36, 37, 56, 190
fruit spreads, 31, 32, 188

G
garlic, 185, 192
G.I. Diet
    and children, 3, 38, 46
    colour-coded food charts, 27–29, 33–35, 37, 38–41, 183–92
    dining out and travel tips, 156–62
    "falling off the wagon", 168
    Phase I and Phase II compared, 20–22
    portions, 25–26
    sample G.I. ratings, 10

shopping list, 193–95
Ten Rules, 196
weekly weight/waist log, 198
gidiet.com, 2, 53
ginger, 102, 123, 127–28, 140
glucose, 6, 9–10, 11, 30, 51, 191. See also sugar
glycemic index, 9–14
grains
    charts, 28, 33, 39, 185
    as part of high-carbohydrate diet, 7
    and processing, 7–9
granola, 28, 185
granola bars,
    homemade, 37, 140, 144
grapefruit, 10, 29, 34, 40, 187–88
grapes, 29, 34, 40, 187
green beans, 34, 40, 93, 107–108, 130, 126–27, 183
green-light ("go ahead") foods, 23
Green-Light Menu Plan, 152–55
grilling, 41, 89
ground beef, 33, 38, 42, 90, 130, 131, 132, 134–35, 136–37, 189
    alternatives to, 42
    extra-lean, 90, 130, 131, 134
    lean, 33, 38, 41, 189
    regular, 33, 38, 189

H
ham (lean), 27, 32, 38, 90, 96, 99
hamburger buns, 184
hamburgers, 33, 38, 189
hash browns, 29, 191
hazelnuts, 29, 37, 40, 187, 190
heart disease,
    and alcohol, 56–57
    and antioxidants, 7
    and cholesterol, 177–78
    and diet, 176–80
    and exercise, 179
    and fats, 4–7
    and risk factors, 19, 51, 61, 164, 171, 176, 181–82
hearts of palm, 192
herbs and spices, 91–92, 186
hot dog buns, 33, 184
hot dogs, 33, 38, 189
hummus, 36, 134, 169, 186
hunger
    and caffeine, 32
    and calories, 20, 21,

noodles, 7, 10, 33, 39, 185, 189
    canned or instant, 33, 39
nut butters, 29, 34, 40, 56, 144, 187
nuts. *See also* specific nuts
    charts, 29, 34, 40, 187
    and protein, 13
    serving sizes, 25, 56, 169
    as snacks, 36, 56, 169
    as source of "good" fat, 5, 46

O
oat bran, 28, 139, 185
oatmeal, 9, 10, 12, 30, 32, 94, 143, 185
    and cholesterol, 12
    and fibre, 12
    and glycemic index, 9, 10
    as "slow-release" food, 9
oats, old-fashioned rolled, 89, 94–95,
    131, 134, 140, 141–42, 143, 144, 146, 185
obesity,
    in adults, 5, 6, 9, 79–80
    and carbohydrates, 14, 82
    in children, 3, 46
    and diabetes, 179
    and fats, 5, 6, 82
    and high blood pressure, 177–78
oils. *See also* fats; specific oils
    comparison chart, 5
    fish, hydrogenated, 6, 42, 46, 181
    monounsaturated ("best"), 5
    polyunsaturated ("better"), 5
    tropical, 29, 35, 40–41, 187
    vegetable, 4, 5, 29, 40, 41, 46, 89, 187
okra, 192
olive oil
    charts, 29, 34, 40, 187
    as cooking oil, 5, 89,
    serving size, 25
olives, 5, 25, 34, 40, 55, 192
omega-3, 6, 42, 181
    eggs, 27, 33, 38, 171, 139–40, 189
onions, 34, 40, 192
oranges, 29, 34, 40, 187, 188
    mandarin, 199
osteoporosis, 171, 181

P
palm oil, 4, 187
pancakes, 28, 33, 184
papayas, 160
parsnips, 34, 40, 191
pasta, 7. *See also* specific pastas
    alfredo, 190

average consumption of, 25
and carbohydrates, 7
charts, 33, 38, 39, 189, 190
cooking al dente, 24, 88
and glycemic index, 24
serving size, 25, 26, 43
whole wheat, 43
pasta sauces, 190
paté, 33, 189
peaches, 29, 34, 40, 85, 188
    canned, 37, 190
peanut butter, 29, 34, 40, 56, 78, 169, 187
peanuts, 5, 29, 34, 187
pears, 34, 40, 106, 149, 188
    canned, 37, 190
peas, 34, 40, 183, 192
penne, 33, 39, 189
peppers
    bell, 34, 36, 40, 191
    green bell, 36
    hot, 34, 40, 192
    red bell, 36
    roasted red, 117
pickles, 34, 37, 40, 190
pita bread, 33, 39, 184
pizza, 33, 39, 78, 112–13, 157, 184
plums, 34, 40, 188
pomegranates, 187
popcorn, 10, 37, 90
pork, 38, 41, 56, 171, 183, 189
    lean cuts, 33, 38
porridge. *See* oatmeal
portions, 25, 90, 158, 167, 169, 196
potato chips, 37, 190
potatoes,
    baked, 10, 24, 34, 40, 192
    boiled, 24, 34, 191
    boiled new, 24, 25, 34, 42, 55, 69,
        93, 161, 192
    french fries, 29, 34, 37, 40, 190, 191
    and glycemic index, 42
    mashed, 34, 40, 192
    serving size, 25
    and starch, 24
poultry, 25, 33, 38, 41–42, 90, 91, 123–29,
    161, 188. *See also* chicken; turkey
pretzels, 37, 190
processed meats, 33, 38
processing of food, 8–9, 13–14, 24
Procrastinator/Avoiders (PAs), 62, 63,
    65, 66, 72
protein
    as brain food, 14

Recipe Index

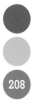